BLACKWELL'S
UNDERGROUND CLINICAL VIGNETTES

NEUROLOGY, 2E

VIKAS BHUSHAN, MD
University of California, San Francisco, Class of 1991
Series Editor, Diagnostic Radiologist

VISHAL PALL, MBBS
Government Medical College, Chandigarh, India, Class of 1996
Series Editor, U. of Texas, Galveston, Resident in Internal Medicine &
Preventive Medicine

TAO LE, MD
University of California, San Francisco, Class of 1996

HOANG NGUYEN, MD, MBA
Northwestern University, Class of 2001

NUTAN SHARMA, MD, PHD
Brigham & Womens Hospital, Fellow in Neurology

D0074339

b

ackwell
cience

CONTRIBUTORS

Fadi Abou-Nukta, MD
University of Damascus, Syria, Class of 1998

Shilpen Patel, MD
University of Maryland, Baltimore, Resident in Radiation Oncology

Kris Alden, MD
University of Illinois, Chicago, MSTP

Sunit Das, MD
Northwestern University, Class of 2000

BLACKWELL'S
UNDERGROUND CLINICAL VIGNETTES

NEUROLOGY, 2E

© 2002 by Blackwell Science, Inc.

Editorial Offices:

Commerce Place, 350 Main Street, Malden,
    Massachusetts 02148, USA
Osney Mead, Oxford OX2 0EL, England
25 John Street, London WC1N 2BS, England
23 Ainslie Place, Edinburgh EH3 6AJ, Scotland
54 University Street, Carlton, Victoria 3053,
    Australia

Other Editorial Offices:

Blackwell Wissenschafts-Verlag GmbH,
    Kurfürstendamm 57, 10707 Berlin, Germany
Blackwell Science KK, MG Kodenmacho Building,
    7-10 Kodenmacho Nihombashi, Chuo-ku,
    Tokyo 104, Japan
Iowa State University Press, A Blackwell Science
    Company, 2121 S. State Avenue, Ames, Iowa
    50014-8300, USA

Distributors:

The Americas
Blackwell Publishing
c/o AIDC
P.O. Box 20
50 Winter Sport Lane
Williston, VT 05495-0020
(Telephone orders: 800-216-2522;
    fax orders: 802-864-7626)
Australia
Blackwell Science Pty, Ltd.
54 University Street
Carlton, Victoria 3053
(Telephone orders: 03-9347-0300;
    fax orders: 03-9349-3016)
Outside The Americas and Australia
Blackwell Science, Ltd.
c/o Marston Book Services, Ltd.
P.O. Box 269
Abingdon
Oxon OX14 4YN
England
(Telephone orders: 44-01235-465500;
    fax orders: 44-01235-465555)

Acquisitions: Laura DeYoung
Development: Amy Nuttbrock
Production: Lorna Hind and Shawn Girsberger
Manufacturing: Lisa Flanagan
Marketing Manager: Kathleen Mulcahy
Cover design by Leslie Haimes
Interior design by Shawn Girsberger
Typeset by TechBooks
Printed and bound by Capital City Press

**Blackwell's Underground Clinical Vignettes:
    Neurology, 2e**
ISBN 0-632-04567-1

Printed in the United States of America
02 03 04 05 5 4 3 2 1

The Blackwell Science logo is a trade mark of
Blackwell Science Ltd., registered at the United
Kingdom Trade Marks Registry

Library of Congress Cataloging-in-Publication Data
Bhushan, Vikas.
Blackwell's underground clinical vignettes.
Neurology / author, Vikas Bhushan. – 2nd ed.
    p. ; cm. – (Underground clinical vignettes) Rev. ed.
of: Neurology / Vikas Bhushan ... [et al.].
c1999. ISBN 0-632-04567-1 (pbk.)
1. Neurology – Case studies. 2. Physicians – Licenses –
United States – Examinations – Study guides.
    [DNLM: 1. Nervous System Diseases –
Case Report. 2. Nervous System Diseases – Problems
and Exercises. WL 18.2 B795b 2002] I. Title:
Underground clinical vignettes. Neurology. II. Title:
Neurology. III. Neurology. IV. Title. V. Series.
    RC359 .B48 2002
    616.8'076–dc21

                                    2001004892

Notice

The authors of this volume have taken care that the information contained herein is accurate and compatible with the standards generally accepted at the time of publication. Nevertheless, it is difficult to ensure that all the information given is entirely accurate for all circumstances. The publisher and authors do not guarantee the contents of this book and disclaim any liability, loss, or damage incurred as a consequence, directly or indirectly, of the use and application of any of the contents of this volume.

CONTENTS

MINICASES

ACKNOWLEDGMENTS

Throughout the production of this book, we have had the support of many friends and colleagues. Special thanks to our support team including Anu Gupta, Andrea Fellows, Anastasia Anderson, Srishti Gupta, Mona Pall, Jonathan Kirsch and Chirag Amin. For prior contributions we thank Gianni Le Nguyen, Tarun Mathur, Alex Grimm, Sonia Santos and Elizabeth Sanders.

We have enjoyed working with a world-class international publishing group at Blackwell Science, including Laura DeYoung, Amy Nuttbrock, Lisa Flanagan, Shawn Girsberger, Lorna Hind and Gordon Tibbitts. For help with securing images for the entire series we also thank Lee Martin, Kristopher Jones, Tina Panizzi and Peter Anderson at the University of Alabama, the Armed Forces Institute of Pathology, and many of our fellow Blackwell Science authors.

For submitting comments, corrections, editing, proofreading, and assistance across all of the vignette titles in all editions, we collectively thank:

Tara Adamovich, Carolyn Alexander, Kris Alden, Henry E. Aryan, Lynman Bacolor, Natalie Barteneva, Dean Bartholomew, Debashish Behera, Sumit Bhatia, Sanjay Bindra, Dave Brinton, Julianne Brown, Alexander Brownie, Tamara Callahan, David Canes, Bryan Casey, Aaron Caughey, Hebert Chen, Jonathan Cheng, Arnold Cheung, Arnold Chin, Simion Chiosea, Yoon Cho, Samuel Chung, Gretchen Conant, Vladimir Coric, Christopher Cosgrove, Ronald Cowan, Karekin R. Cunningham, A. Sean Dalley, Rama Dandamudi, Sunit Das, Ryan Armando Dave, John David, Emmanuel de la Cruz, Robert DeMello, Navneet Dhillon, Sharmila Dissanaike, David Donson, Adolf Etchegaray, Alea Eusebio, Priscilla A. Frase, David Frenz, Kristin Gaumer, Yohannes Gebreegziabher, Anil Gehi, Tony George, L.M. Gotanco, Parul Goyal, Alex Grimm, Rajeev Gupta, Ahmad Halim, Sue Hall, David Hasselbacher, Tamra Heimert, Michelle Higley, Dan Hoit, Eric Jackson, Tim Jackson, Sundar Jayaraman, Pei-Ni Jone, Aarchan Joshi, Rajni K. Jutla, Faiyaz Kapadi, Seth Karp, Aaron S. Kesselheim, Sana Khan, Andrew Pin-wei Ko, Francis Kong, Paul Konitzky, Warren S. Krackov, Benjamin H.S. Lau, Ann LaCasce, Connie Lee, Scott Lee, Guillermo Lehmann, Kevin Leung, Paul Levett, Warren Levinson, Eric Ley, Ken Lin,

Pavel Lobanov, J. Mark Maddox, Aram Mardian, Samir Mehta,
Gil Melmed, Joe Messina, Robert Mosca, Michael Murphy, Vivek
Nandkarni, Siva Naraynan, Carvell Nguyen, Linh Nguyen,
Deanna Nobleza, Craig Nodurft, George Noumi, Darin T.
Okuda, Adam L. Palance, Paul Pamphrus, Jinha Park, Sonny
Patel, Ricardo Pietrobon, Riva L. Rahl, Aashita Randeria,
Rachan Reddy, Beatriu Reig, Marilou Reyes, Jeremy Richmon,
Tai Roe, Rick Roller, Rajiv Roy, Diego Ruiz, Anthony Russell,
Sanjay Sahgal, Urmimala Sarkar, John Schilling, Isabell Schmitt,
Daren Schuhmacher, Sonal Shah, Edie Shen, Justin Smith, John
Stulak, Lillian Su, Julie Sundaram, Rita Suri, Seth Sweetser,
Antonio Talayero, Merita Tan, Mark Tanaka, Eric Taylor, Jess
Thompson, Indi Trehan, Raymond Turner, Okafo Uchenna,
Eric Uyguanco, Richa Varma, John Wages, Alan Wang, Eunice
Wang, Andy Weiss, Amy Williams, Brian Yang, Hany Zaky, Ashraf
Zaman and David Zipf.

For generously contributing images to the entire *Underground
Clinical Vignette* Step 2 series, we collectively thank the staff at
Blackwell Science in Oxford, Boston, and Berlin as well as:

- Alfred Cuschieri, Thomas P.J. Hennessy, Roger M.
  Greenhalgh, David I. Rowley, Pierce A. Grace (*Clinical
  Surgery*, © 1996 Blackwell Science), Figures 13.23, 13.35b,
  13.51, 15.13, 15.2.

- John Axford (*Medicine*, © 1996 Blackwell Science), Figures
  f3.10, 2.103a, 2.110b, 3.20a, 3.20b, 3.25b, 3.38a, 5.9Bi, 5.9Bii,
  6.41a, 6.41b, 6.74b, 6.74c, 7.78ai, 7.78aii, 7.78b, 8.47b, 9.9e,
  f3.17, f3.36, f3.37, f5.27, f5.28, f5.45a, f5.48, f5.49a, f5.50,
  f5.65a, f5.67, f5.68, f8.27a, 10.120b, 11.63b, 11.63c, 11.68a,
  11.68b, 11.68c, 12.37a, 12.37b.

- Peter Armstrong, Martin L. Wastie (*Diagnostic Imaging*, 4th
  Edition, © 1998 Blackwell Science), Figures 2.100, 2.108d,
  2.109, 2.11, 2.112, 2.121, 2.122, 2.13, 2.1ba, 2.1bb, 2.36, 2.53,
  2.54, 2.69a, 2.71, 2.80a, 2.81b, 2.82, 2.84a, 2.84b, 2.88, 2.89a,
  2.89b, 2.90b, 2.94a, 2.94b, 2.96, 2.97, 2.98a, 2.98c, 3.11, 3.19,
  3.20, 3.21, 3.22, 3.28, 3.30, 3.34, 3.35b, 3.35c, 3.36, 4.7, 4.8,
  4.9, 5.29, 5.33, 5.58, 5.62, 5.63, 5.64, 5.65b, 5.66a, 5.66b, 5.69,
  5.71, 5.75, 5.8, 5.9, 6.17a, 6.17b, 6.25, 6.28, 6.29c, 6.30, 7.13,
  7.17a, 7.45a, 7.45b, 7.46, 7.50, 7.52, 7.53a, 7.57a, 7.58, 8.7a,
  8.7b, 8.7c, 8.86, 8.8a, 8.96, 8.9a, 9.17a, 9.17b, 10.13a, 10.13b,
  10.14a, 10.14b, 10.14c, 10.17a, 10.17b, 11.16b, 11.17a, 11.17b,
  11.19, 11.23, 11.24, 11.2b, 11.2d, 11.30a, 11.30b, 12.12, 12.15,

12.18, 12.19, 12.3, 12.4, 12.8a, 12.8b, 13.13a, 13.18, 13.18a, 13.20, 13.22a, 13.22b, 13.29, 14.14a, 14.5, 14.6a, 15.25b, 15.29b, 15.31, 15.37, 17.4.

- N.C. Hughes-Jones, S.N. Wickramasinghe (*Lecture Notes On: Haematology, 6th Edition*, © 1996 Blackwell Science), Figures 2.1b, 2.2a, 3.14, 3.8, 4.3, 5.2b, 5.5a, 5.8, 7.1, 7.2, 7.3, 7.5, 8.1, 10.5b, 10.6, 11.1, plate 29, plate 34, plate 44, plate 45, plate 48, plate 5, plate 42.

- Thomas Grumme, Wolfgang Kluge, Konrad Kretzschmar, Andreas Roesler (*Cerebral and Spinal Computed Tomography, 3rd Edition*, © 1998 Blackwell Science), Figures 16.2b, 16.3, 16.6a, 17.1a, 18-1c, 18-5, 41.3c, 41.3d, 44.3, 46.8, 47.7, 48.2, 48.6a, 53.5, 55.2a, 55.2c, 56.2b, 57.1, 61.3a, 61.3b, 63.1a, 64.3a, 65.3c, 66.3b, 67.6, 70.1a, 70.3, 81.2a, 81.4, 82.2, 82.3, 84.6.

- P.R. Patel (*Lecture Notes On: Radiology*, © 1998 Blackwell Science), Figures 2.15, 2.16, 2.25, 2.26, 2.30, 2.31, 2.33, 2.36, 3.11, 3.16, 3.19, 3.4, 3.7, 4.19, 4.20, 4.38, 4.44, 4.45, 4.46, 4.47, 4.49, 4.5, 5.14, 5.6, 6.18, 6.19, 6.20, 6.21, 6.22, 6.31a, 6.31b, 7.18, 7.19, 7.21, 7.22, 7.32, 7.34, 7.41, 7.46a, 7.46b, 7.48, 7.49, 7.9, 8.2, 8.3, 8.4, 8.5, 8.8, 8.9, 9.12, 9.2, 9.3, 9.8, 9.9, 10.11, 10.16, 10.5.

- Ramsay Vallance (*An Atlas of Diagnostic Radiology in Gastroenterology*, © 1999 Blackwell Science), Figures 1.22, 2.57, 2.27, 2.55a, 2.58, 2.59, 2.63, 2.64, 2.65, 3.11, 3.3, 3.37, 3.39, 3.4, 4.6a, 4.8, 4.9, 5.1, 5.29, 5.63, 5.64b, 5.65b, 5.66b, 5.68a, 5.68b, 6.110, 6.15, 6.17, 6.23, 6.29b, 6.30, 6.39, 6.64a, 6.64b, 6.75, 6.78, 6.80, 7.57a, 7.57c, 7.60a, 8.17, 8.48, 8.53, 8.66, 9.11a, 9.15, 9.17, 9.23, 9.24, 9.25, 9.28, 9.30, 9.32a, 9.33, 9.43, 9.45, 9.55b, 9.57, 9.63, 9.64a, 9.64b, 9.64c, 9.66, 10.28, 10.36, 10.44, 10.6.

Please let us know if your name has been missed or misspelled and we will be happy to make the update in the next edition.

PREFACE TO THE 2ND EDITION

We were very pleased with the overwhelmingly positive student feedback for the 1st edition of our *Underground Clinical Vignettes* series. Well over 100,000 copies of the UCV books are in print and have been used by students all over the world.

Over the last two years we have accumulated and incorporated **over a thousand "updates"** and improvements suggested by you, our readers, including:

• many additions of specific boards and wards testable content

• deletions of redundant and overlapping cases

• reordering and reorganization of all cases in both series

• a new master index by case name in each Atlas

• correction of a few factual errors

• diagnosis and treatment updates

• addition of 5–20 new cases in every book

• and the addition of clinical exam photographs within *UCV—Anatomy*

And most important of all, the second edition sets now include two brand new **COLOR ATLAS** supplements, one for each Clinical Vignette series.

• The *UCV–Basic Science Color Atlas* (*Step 1*) includes over 250 color plates, divided into gross pathology, microscopic pathology (histology), hematology, and microbiology (smears).

• The *UCV–Clinical Science Color Atlas* (*Step 2*) has over 125 color plates, including patient images, dermatology, and funduscopy.

Each atlas image is descriptively captioned and linked to its corresponding Step 1 case, Step 2 case, and/or Step 2 MiniCase.

How Atlas Links Work:

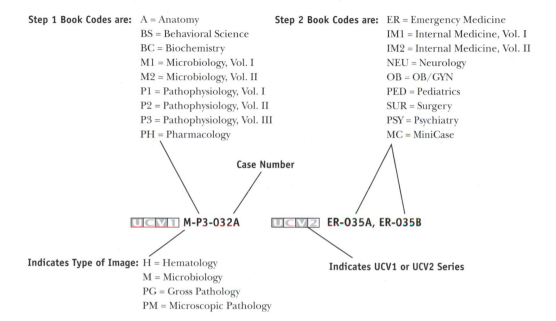

Step 1 Book Codes are:
A = Anatomy
BS = Behavioral Science
BC = Biochemistry
M1 = Microbiology, Vol. I
M2 = Microbiology, Vol. II
P1 = Pathophysiology, Vol. I
P2 = Pathophysiology, Vol. II
P3 = Pathophysiology, Vol. III
PH = Pharmacology

Step 2 Book Codes are:
ER = Emergency Medicine
IM1 = Internal Medicine, Vol. I
IM2 = Internal Medicine, Vol. II
NEU = Neurology
OB = OB/GYN
PED = Pediatrics
SUR = Surgery
PSY = Psychiatry
MC = MiniCase

Case Number

UCV1 M-P3-032A   UCV2 ER-035A, ER-035B

Indicates Type of Image:
H = Hematology
M = Microbiology
PG = Gross Pathology
PM = Microscopic Pathology

Indicates UCV1 or UCV2 Series

- If the Case number (032, 035, etc.) is not followed by a letter, then there is only one image. Otherwise A, B, C, D indicate up to 4 images.

Bold Faced Links: In order to give you access to the largest number of images possible, we have chosen to cross link the Step 1 and 2 series.

- If the link is bold-faced this indicates that the link is direct (i.e., Step 1 Case with the Basic Science Step 1 Atlas link).

- If the link is not bold-faced this indicates that the link is indirect (Step 1 case with Clinical Science Step 2 Atlas link or vice versa).

We have also implemented a few structural changes upon your request:

- Each current and future edition of our popular *First Aid for the USMLE Step 1* (Appleton & Lange/McGraw-Hill) and *First Aid for the USMLE Step 2* (Appleton & Lange/McGraw-Hill) book will be linked to the corresponding UCV case.

- We eliminated UCV → First Aid links as they frequently become out of date, as the *First Aid* books are revised yearly.

- The Color Atlas is also specially designed for quizzing—captions are descriptive and do not give away the case name directly.

New "MiniCases" replace the previous "Associated Diseases." There are now over **350 unique MiniCases** distributed throughout the *Step 2 Clinical* series, selected based on recent USMLE recollections.

We hope the updated UCV series will remain a unique and well-integrated study tool that provides compact clinical correlations to basic science information. They are designed to be easy and fun (comparatively) to read, and helpful for both licensing exams and the wards.

We invite your corrections and suggestions for the fourth edition of these books. For the first submission of each factual correction or new vignette that is selected for inclusion in the fourth edition, you will receive a personal acknowledgment in the revised book. If you submit over 20 high-quality corrections, additions or new vignettes we will also consider **inviting you to become a "Contributor" on the book of your choice**. If you are interested in becoming a potential "Contributor" or "Author" on a future UCV book, or working with our team in developing additional books, please also e-mail us your CV/resume.

We prefer that you submit corrections or suggestions via electronic mail to **UCVteam@yahoo.com**. Please include "Underground Vignettes" as the subject of your message. If you do not have access to e-mail, use the following mailing address: Blackwell Publishing, Attn: UCV Editors, 350 Main Street, Malden, MA 02148, USA.

Vikas Bhushan
Vishal Pall
Tao Le
October 2001

This series was originally developed to address the increasing number of clinical vignette questions on medical examinations, including the USMLE Step 1 and Step 2. It is also designed to supplement and complement the popular *First Aid for the USMLE Step 1* (Appleton & Lange/McGraw Hill) and *First Aid for the USMLE Step 2* (Appleton & Lange/McGraw Hill).

Each UCV 2 book uses a series of approximately 50 **"supra-prototypical" cases as a way to condense testable facts and associations**. The clinical vignettes in this series are designed to give added emphasis to pathogenesis, epidemiology, management and complications. They also contain relevant extensive B/W imaging plates within each book. Additionally, each UCV2 book contains approximately 30 to 60 "MiniCases" that focus on presenting only the key facts for that disease in a tightly edited fashion.

Although each case tends to present all the signs, symptoms, and diagnostic findings for a particular illness, **patients generally will not present with such a "complete" picture either clinically or on a medical examination**. Cases are not meant to simulate a potential real patient or an exam vignette. All the **boldfaced "buzzwords" are for learning purposes** and are not necessarily expected to be found in any one patient with the disease.

Definitions of selected important terms are placed within the vignettes in (SMALL CAPS) in parentheses. Other parenthetical remarks often refer to the pathophysiology or mechanism of disease. The format should also help students learn to present cases succinctly during oral "bullet" presentations on clinical rotations. The cases are meant to serve as a condensed review, not as a primary reference. The information provided in this book has been prepared with a great deal of thought and careful research. This book should not, however, be considered as your sole source of information. Corrections, suggestions and submissions of new cases are encouraged and will be acknowledged and incorporated when appropriate in future editions.

ABBREVIATIONS

5-ASA	5-aminosalicylic acid
ABGs	arterial blood gases
ABVD	adriamycin/bleomycin/vincristine/dacarbazine
ACE	angiotensin-converting enzyme
ACTH	adrenocorticotropic hormone
ADH	antidiuretic hormone
AFP	alpha fetal protein
AI	aortic insufficiency
AIDS	acquired immunodeficiency syndrome
ALL	acute lymphocytic leukemia
ALT	alanine transaminase
AML	acute myelogenous leukemia
ANA	antinuclear antibody
ARDS	adult respiratory distress syndrome
ASD	atrial septal defect
ASO	anti-streptolysin O
AST	aspartate transaminase
AV	arteriovenous
BE	barium enema
BP	blood pressure
BUN	blood urea nitrogen
CAD	coronary artery disease
CALLA	common acute lymphoblastic leukemia antigen
CBC	complete blood count
CHF	congestive heart failure
CK	creatine kinase
CLL	chronic lymphocytic leukemia
CML	chronic myelogenous leukemia
CMV	cytomegalovirus
CNS	central nervous system
COPD	chronic obstructive pulmonary disease
CPK	creatine phosphokinase
CSF	cerebrospinal fluid
CT	computed tomography
CVA	cerebrovascular accident
CXR	chest x-ray
DIC	disseminated intravascular coagulation
DIP	distal interphalangeal
DKA	diabetic ketoacidosis
DM	diabetes mellitus
DTRs	deep tendon reflexes
DVT	deep venous thrombosis

EBV	Epstein–Barr virus
ECG	electrocardiography
Echo	echocardiography
EF	ejection fraction
EGD	esophagogastroduodenoscopy
EMG	electromyography
ERCP	endoscopic retrograde cholangiopancreatography
ESR	erythrocyte sedimentation rate
FEV	forced expiratory volume
FNA	fine needle aspiration
FTA-ABS	fluorescent treponemal antibody absorption
FVC	forced vital capacity
GFR	glomerular filtration rate
GH	growth hormone
GI	gastrointestinal
GM-CSF	granulocyte macrophage colony stimulating factor
GU	genitourinary
HAV	hepatitis A virus
hcG	human chorionic gonadotrophin
HEENT	head, eyes, ears, nose, and throat
HIV	human immunodeficiency virus
HLA	human leukocyte antigen
HPI	history of present illness
HR	heart rate
HRIG	human rabies immune globulin
HS	hereditary spherocytosis
ID/CC	identification and chief complaint
IDDM	insulin-dependent diabetes mellitus
Ig	immunoglobulin
IGF	insulin-like growth factor
IM	intramuscular
JVP	jugular venous pressure
KUB	kidneys/ureter/bladder
LDH	lactate dehydrogenase
LES	lower esophageal sphincter
LFTs	liver function tests
LP	lumbar puncture
LV	left ventricular
LVH	left ventricular hypertrophy
Lytes	electrolytes
MCHC	mean corpuscular hemoglobin concentration
MCV	mean corpuscular volume
MEN	multiple endocrine neoplasia

MGUS	monoclonal gammopathy of undetermined significance
MHC	major histocompatibility complex
MI	myocardial infarction
MOPP	mechlorethamine/vincristine (Oncovorin)/procarbazine/prednisone
MR	magnetic resonance (imaging)
NHL	non-Hodgkin's lymphoma
NIDDM	non-insulin-dependent diabetes mellitus
NPO	nil per os (nothing by mouth)
NSAID	nonsteroidal anti-inflammatory drug
PA	posteroanterior
PIP	proximal interphalangeal
PBS	peripheral blood smear
PE	physical exam
PFTs	pulmonary function tests
PMI	point of maximal intensity
PMN	polymorphonuclear leukocyte
PT	prothrombin time
PTCA	percutaneous transluminal angioplasty
PTH	parathyroid hormone
PTT	partial thromboplastin time
PUD	peptic ulcer disease
RBC	red blood cell
RPR	rapid plasma reagin
RR	respiratory rate
RS	Reed–Sternberg (cell)
RV	right ventricular
RVH	right ventricular hypertrophy
SBFT	small bowel follow-through
SIADH	syndrome of inappropriate secretion of ADH
SLE	systemic lupus erythematosus
STD	sexually transmitted disease
TFTs	thyroid function tests
tPA	tissue plasminogen activator
TSH	thyroid-stimulating hormone
TIBC	total iron-binding capacity
TIPS	transjugular intrahepatic portosystemic shunt
TPO	thyroid peroxidase
TSH	thyroid-stimulating hormone
TTP	thrombotic thrombocytopenic purpura
UA	urinalysis
UGI	upper GI
US	ultrasound

VDRL	Venereal Disease Research Laboratory
VS	vital signs
VT	ventricular tachycardia
WBC	white blood cell
WPW	Wolff–Parkinson–White (syndrome)
XR	x-ray

ID/CC   A **45-year-old male** complains of slowly **progressive muscle weakness** involving the **hands and lower limbs**.

HPI   He has had muscle wasting, weakness, rigidity, and slowness. He denies any incontinence or changes in his bowel habits. He has also noted difficulty walking (impaired gait).

PE   VS: normal. PE: **muscle atrophy**, weakness, wasting, **fasciculations**, loss of stretch reflexes, and bradykinesia noted in **upper extremities** bilaterally (LMN signs); **muscle rigidity, spasticity**, clonus, and hyperactive DTRs noted in bilateral **lower extremities** (UMN signs); **Babinski's present** (UMN sign); spastic gait; no sensory deficit.

Labs   Muscle biopsy shows **grouping of muscle fiber types** (as nerves die, adjacent nerves send buds to reinnervate muscle and fibers switch types). LP: mildly elevated protein (50 mg/dL) in CSF. EMG: **fasciculations** and evidence of **denervation** in upper extremities with **normal nerve conduction velocities**.

Imaging   CT/MR, brain and spinal cord: normal.

Pathogenesis   Amyotrophic lateral sclerosis (ALS) is also known as **Lou Gehrig's disease**. The cause is unknown; it is usually sporadic and associated with an infectious etiology. Affects both **anterior horn cells** in the spinal cord and **UMNs** in the corticospinal tract, resulting in both UMN and LMN deficits. UMN and LMN signs may be asymmetric.

Epidemiology   **Males** are more likely to be affected than females. **Incidence rises after age 40** and continues to increase until about 80. Occasionally associated with dementia and parkinsonism. A familial form of the disease with autosomal-dominant inheritance has been identified.

Management   **No specific treatment. Riluzole**, which reduces the presynaptic release of glutamate, may slow progression. Symptomatic management is indicated, including anticholinergics to prevent drooling and braces and physical therapy to assist mobility and prevent contractures.

Complications   Dysphagia, respiratory compromise, and aspiration; **death within 5 years of symptom onset**.

AMYOTROPHIC LATERAL SCLEROSIS (ALS)

ID/CC	A **10-year-old** male presents with a **severe headache** that does not respond to analgesics, along with **projectile vomiting**.
HPI	In the ER, he suffered a **seizure**. The headache was present upon awakening. Directed questioning reveals that he has been behaving oddly for the past month.
PE	VS: normal. PE: appears confused; **ataxic gait; bilateral papilledema** and **nystagmus**; mild hypotonia of left arm; cardiopulmonary and abdominal exams normal.
Labs	CBC: normal. SaO_2 99%. Lytes: normal. UA: normal. LP/LFTs: normal. TFTs: normal.
Imaging	**[A]** CT, head: enhancing, irregular **cerebellar mass** (1) with cystic areas in the left posterior cranial fossa. **[B]** MR, brain (sagittal): another posterior fossa enhancing astrocytoma.
Pathogenesis	Astrocytomas are **slow-growing** (with the exception of grade 4 astrocytoma, or glioblastoma multiforme), **malignant brain tumors** that **originate from neuroectodermal neuroglia**; in **children** they are usually **located in the cerebellum**, whereas in adults they are located in the cerebrum. Astrocytomas are commonly cystic in children, and their growth may cause increased ICP, seizures, and hydrocephalus.
Epidemiology	Brain tumors are the second most common cause of childhood cancer and the **most common solid tumors in childhood** (followed by medulloblastoma and ependymoma). There is a higher incidence of astrocytomas in children with previous CNS irradiation, neurofibromatosis, and tuberous sclerosis as well as in children with a family history. Age < 4 years is an unfavorable prognostic sign.

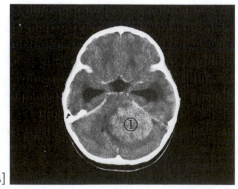

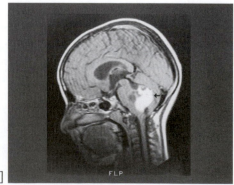

[A] [B]

ASTROCYTOMA

Management Stage the disease with CSF analysis, MRI, and angiography if necessary. **Dexamethasone** is used to decrease brain edema, and **phenytoin** is used as an anticonvulsant. **Surgical resection** depends on the location of the tumor. Most patients will eventually need radiation. Chemotherapy may temporarily control the disease, allowing radiotherapy to be postponed to a later age, when outcomes are better.

Complications **Hydrocephalus, seizures**, herniation, functional loss, and irradiation damage (neuropsychological disturbances, hypothyroidism, growth retardation).

Atlas Link   UCVI PG-A-052

MINICASE 231: RABIES

Caused by an infection of the CNS by rhabdovirus (a single-stranded, enveloped, RNA virus) that is transmitted to humans by the bites of skunks, raccoons, foxes, and bats or, rarely, by corneal transplants
- presents with fever, paresthesias, muscle spasms, confusion, hydrophobia, convulsions, and increased lacrimation
- positive titers of neutralizing antibody to rabies, positive rabies antigen in corneal smears, brain biopsy reveals Negri bodies
- treat supportively (respiratory, circulatory, and CNS)
- pre- and postexposure prophylaxis is available with rabies immune globulin and/or human diploid cell vaccine
- death usually results from respiratory failure

Atlas Link: UCVI M-M2-041

MINICASE 232: TETANUS

A neurologic syndrome caused by a neurotoxin (tetanospasmin) produced by *Clostridium tetani* (an anaerobic, spore-forming, gram-positive rod)
- the usual portals of entry are traumatic wounds, surgical wounds, or subcutaneous injection sites
- presents with grimacing, painful muscular contractions (usually of the jaw and neck), opisthotonos, dysphagia, or seizures
- treat with surgical debridement of the wound and supportive care (intubation or tracheostomy for laryngospasm, diazepam to control muscle spasms), tetanus immune globulin, tetanus toxoid, and penicillin

Atlas Link: UCVI M-M2-062

ID/CC	A 45-year-old female presents with new-onset right-sided **facial weakness** and **drooping of the right side of the mouth**.
HPI	She complains of a sore right eye (due to drying of the cornea). She also becomes irritated upon hearing even minor noises, complaining that they are "too loud" (HYPERACUSIS).
PE	Alert and oriented ×3; funduscopy normal; right-sided **paralysis of upper and lower face** such that eye cannot be closed tightly (or can easily be opened by physician); eyeball turns up on attempted closure (BELL'S PHENOMENON); patient is **unable to raise right eyebrow** (LOWER MOTOR NEURON RIGHT FACIAL PALSY); corner of mouth droops and **nasolabial fold** is **decreased**; voluntary and involuntary movements of mouth are paralyzed on right side (lips are drawn to opposite side); examination of right ear normal (to rule out herpetic Ramsay Hunt syndrome); no other cranial nerve palsy found; no other neurologic deficit.
Imaging	CT, head: no intracranial lesions or hemorrhage.
Pathogenesis	Bell's palsy is by definition **idiopathic**. Approximately 80% of patients recover fully.
Epidemiology	The **most common form of facial paralysis**.
Management	**No specific treatment**. Artificial tears and taping the eye shut at night. High-dose corticosteroids may shorten the disease course.
Complications	Chronic paralysis in a minority of cases.

MINICASE 233: APHASIA—CONDUCTION

Disconnection between language centers due to a temporal lobe lesion
- presents with fluent, paraphasic speech that is incomprehensible
- receptive comprehension intact
- CT or MR reveals lesion of the temporal lobe
- treat with speech therapy

ID/CC   A 17-year-old male who was **stabbed in the back** presents with
         inability to use his left leg along with stiffness and **loss of pain
         sensation in the right leg**.

HPI   The stab wound extended to the spinal cord at the level of L1
         slightly to the left of the spinous process. Since the injury, the
         patient has been unable to move his left leg. He also complains
         of episodes of "tingling" of the distal left leg.

PE   VS: normal. PE: cranial nerves intact; motor exam demonstrates
         5/5 strength bilaterally in upper extremities, 5/5 strength in
         right lower extremity, and 0/5 strength in left lower extremity;
         increased tone in left leg; DTRs 2+ and symmetric in upper
         extremities, 3+ in left patella and Achilles, and 2+ in right
         patella and Achilles; **diminished proprioception and vibration
         sense** in left leg; **loss of pain and temperature** sense in right leg;
         Babinski's present in left leg.

Imaging MR, spine: no intramedullary mass identified.

Pathogenesis   Brown-Séquard syndrome is due to **hemisection of the spinal
               cord**. This results in ipsilateral UMN signs below the lesion
               (hyperreflexia, spastic paralysis resulting from lateral corti-
               cospinal tract interruption), ipsilateral loss of vibration and pro-
               prioception sense (due to damage to the dorsal column), and
               contralateral loss of pain and temperature sensation (due to
               damage of the spinothalamic tract that decussated below lesion).

Epidemiology   Typically occurs secondary to **trauma** (e.g., bullet or stab
               wounds), spinal cord **tumor**, or fracture-dislocation causing
               compression.

Management   **Symptomatic relief** of hyperesthesias; phenytoin and carba-
               mazepine are effective.

Complications Limited mobility may result in pressure ulcers or URIs; the neu-
               rologic syndrome itself does not progress.

BROWN-SÉQUARD SYNDROME

ID/CC A 4-year-old female who was **born prematurely** presents with **difficulty walking**.

HPI The child was born after a difficult delivery, at 28 weeks. Almost all developmental milestones (especially motor) were delayed and she has learned to walk only within the past year. Her parents have noted that her **gait is clumsy and stiff** (SPASTIC GAIT). She also has abnormal, **abrupt, jerky movements of her limbs** (CHOREA) and sometimes **slow, writhing, continuous movements** (ATHETOSIS).

PE Motor strength 4/5 in both lower extremities and 5/5 in both upper extremities; **motor tone increased** in lower extremities but normal in upper extremities; DTRs 3+ bilaterally in lower extremities and 2+ bilaterally in upper extremities; **Moro's and asymmetrical tonic neck reflexes persist**.

Imaging MR, brain: **periventricular white matter disease**.

Pathogenesis Cerebral palsy is a motor deficit of **unknown etiology** due to a nonprogressive lesion in the immature brain. The pathology may occur at any stage of brain development. Premature newborns may suffer from periventricular hemorrhage affecting the white matter, which primarily carries that portion of the corticospinal tract which is responsible for leg movement.

Epidemiology Cerebral palsy is associated with **cerebral anoxia** at birth, **prematurity, trauma, embryologic malformations**, and **infection**.

Management **Physical and occupational therapy** should be initiated at birth. Orthotic devices should be used if ambulation is significantly affected. Treat associated problems such as seizures and learning disabilities.

Complications Complications depend on the severity of cerebral palsy. If mobility is severely limited, patients may suffer from pneumonia, UTIs, and decubitus ulcers. Associated problems include epilepsy, mental retardation, behavioral problems, and learning disabilities.

Atlas Link ⊔C⊽2 NEU-005

ID/CC A **26-year-old male** complains of having **"terrible headaches"** for the past 5 years.

HPI The headaches usually occur at night and generally start with a **burning in the right eye** that, within minutes, involves the right orbit and right temple. The pain feels like a "hot poker" behind the right eye; the right eye then starts **tearing** and the **right nostril begins to run**. The pain lasts for 45 minutes. The patient generally has **three to four attacks within a 24-hour period every 6 months**. He states that the **symptoms usually occur after** consumption of **alcohol**.

PE VS: normal. PE: neurologic exam normal; **lacrimation** from right eye; during an acute episode, ptosis, miosis, anhidrosis, and enophthalmos of the right eye are present (HORNER'S SYNDROME).

Labs CBC: normal. ESR: normal.

Imaging MR/CT, brain: no intracranial lesion or hemorrhage; no significant abnormality.

Pathogenesis The pathology of cluster headache is thought to be vascular in nature. The neurotransmitter **substance P** may mediate the pain.

Epidemiology Cluster headaches usually occur in **patients in their 20s** and are much more common in **males**. Many patients report that attacks **occur at the same time of year** (e.g., January and July).

Management Prophylactic treatment consists of **verapamil** or **methysergide** for 1 to 2 months (methysergide should not be prescribed for longer periods owing to the risk of retroperitoneal fibrosis). **Prednisone, ergotamine**, and **lithium** are also used for prophylactic treatment. **Abortive therapy** consists of **100% high-flow oxygen** at 8 to 10 L/min, **intranasal lidocaine**, or **sumatriptan**.

Complications Recurrence and persistence into late life.

CLUSTER HEADACHE

ID/CC	A 16-year-old boy presents with **short stature** and **delayed onset of puberty**.
HPI	He also complains of **intolerance to cold, easy fatigability, dry skin**, and **constipation**. Directed questioning reveals that he has also been suffering from **polyuria**.
PE	VS: normal. PE: short for age; papilledema and optic disk swelling (due to increased ICP) as well as **bitemporal hemianopsia** (due to impingement on optic chiasm).
Labs	CBC: normal. Low T_3, T_4, and TSH. Lytes: hypernatremia. UA: low specific gravity (< 1.006) (due to diabetes insipidus).
Imaging	**[A]** CT, head: small, calcified suprasellar mass. **[B]** CT, head (contrast): large cystic craniopharyngioma. MR: classically, an enhancing **cystic, multilobulated suprasellar mass with ring calcification**; hydrocephalus (due to obstruction of foramen of Munro and aqueduct of Sylvius).
Pathogenesis	Craniopharyngioma is a tumor that is embryologically derived from squamous cell **remnants of Rathke's pouch**. It is usually located in the **suprasellar region** and **causes growth retardation, diabetes insipidus** (due to compression of the pituitary), **bitemporal hemianopsia** (due to pressure on the optic chiasm), and **headache** (due to obstructive hydrocephalus). The clinical significance of this **histologically benign** tumor lies in its proximity to the optic chiasm, the carotid arteries, CN III, and the pituitary stalk.
Epidemiology	The **most common supratentorial brain tumor in children**; has a bimodal age distribution with a second peak in incidence in the fifth decade of life.

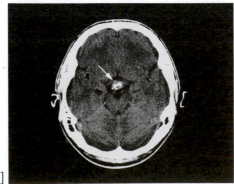

[A]

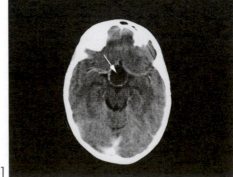

[B]

Management	**Needle aspiration** has the lowest morbidity but is associated with a higher recurrence rate. **Surgical resection** of as much tumor as possible without endangering the endocrine and intellectual functions is the usual treatment. Radiation is always needed after aspiration and sometimes after surgical excision. Hydrocortisone is usually given in the perioperative period.
Complications	Necrosis of the pituitary stalk during surgery with release of ADH and a sharp decrease in urinary volume; postoperative recurrence of tumor.
Atlas Link	ⓊⒸⓋⓉ PG-P3-006

MINICASE 234: BRAIN ABSCESS

A focal intracerebral infection beginning as a localized area of cerebritis and progressing to a collection of pus surrounded by a well-vascularized capsule

- abscesses usually arise either from contiguous infection (e.g., paranasal sinuses infecting the frontal lobe, otitis media/mastoiditis infecting the temporal lobe or cerebellum, dental sepsis infecting the frontal lobes, or penetrating head injury/postneurosurgical procedures) or from hematogenous spread (e.g., congenital heart disease, infective endocarditis, bronchiectasis/lung abscesses, or immune-compromised states associated with opportunistic infections)
- the most common organisms include streptococci, staphylococci, anaerobes, and *Toxoplasma* or fungi in immune-compromised patients
- presents with headache, drowsiness, confusion, and seizures
- lumbar puncture is contraindicated, MR/CT scan shows a contrast-enhanced, ringlike mass with surrounding edema
- treat with IV antibiotics combined with surgical drainage
- complications include focal neurologic deficits and increased intracranial pressure

---

MINICASE 235: CARBAMAZEPINE TOXICITY

Due to overdosage, use of usual doses in liver disease, or concomitant use of drugs that increase serum levels (erythromycin, cimetidine, and isoniazid)

- presents with respiratory depression, coma, tremors, arrhythmia, marked fluctuations in blood pressure, and mydriasis
- serum levels elevated ($>$ 20 mg/mL)
- treat with gastric lavage, hemoperfusion
- other side effects include idiosyncratic leukopenia, aplastic anemia, Stevens-Johnson syndrome, and toxic epidermal necrolysis

ID/CC	A **60-year-old** male presents with a rapidly progressive **change in mental status** over the past 2 months with an **inability to concentrate** and **memory impairment**.
HPI	His relatives have noticed increased somnolence, changes in his personality, and **twitching movements of the hands** and **difficulty walking** (due to ataxia) for several months.
PE	VS: normal. PE: no papilledema; normal speech; **ataxic gait** with **choreoathetotic movements** and **myoclonus**; normal DTRs; normal sensation; cranial nerves intact.
Labs	CBC/Lytes: normal. TFTs: normal. LFTs: normal. LP: CSF analysis normal. EEG: **diffuse, slow background with superimposed bilateral sharp triphasic synchronous discharge complexes**.
Imaging	CT/MR, brain: generalized cortical atrophy.
Pathogenesis	Creutzfeldt–Jakob disease (CJD) is a **subacute encephalopathy of the spongiform type** that is caused by a slow-virus-like agent (PRION) with a very long incubation period. CJD gives rise to progressive dementia and associated myoclonus and may be **transmitted** by **corneal transplants, dura mater allografts**, contaminated **cadaveric growth hormone, EEG electrodes**, and **neurosurgical contamination**. Pathologic findings include softening of CNS tissue with vacuolization and secondary amyloidosis but no inflammatory reaction. Unlike Alzheimer's, there is very little cerebral atrophy owing to the rapid progression of the disease. CJD is diagnosed by brain biopsy after other causes of dementia have been ruled out.
Epidemiology	Occurs with greater frequency in the sixth decade of life; shows no gender predominance. Has a higher incidence within families and in certain geographical areas, such as Czechoslovakia, North Africa, and Chile. Between 5% and 15% of cases are autosomal dominant. Closely associated with **kuru from New Guinea**, which is now a rare disease (was transmitted by some tribal traditions of eating human brains). The disease **progresses rapidly**; 1-year survival is rare.
Management	**No specific treatment is available**, and the disease has a very **poor short-term prognosis**.
Complications	Coma and death.

ID/CC An **82-year-old** woman with known dementia who resides at a nursing home presents with a change in mental status.

HPI The patient was in her usual state of health at dinner the previous night. In the morning, she complained of headache and could not move her right arm.

PE VS: no fever; **hypertension** (BP 160/95). PE: drowsy but able to follow simple commands; right facial droop noted; 0/5 strength in right arm and 4/5 strength in right leg; 5/5 strength in left arm and leg; DTRs 2+ in left arm and leg and **3+ in right arm and leg**; Babinski's absent.

Labs CBC/Lytes: normal. PT/PTT, glucose, BUN, and creatinine normal.

Imaging [A] CT, head: cortical hemorrhage in the left frontal lobe (1).

Pathogenesis Cerebral amyloid angiopathy (CAA) is characterized by **deposition of amyloid in small and medium-sized arteries in the cortex**. It may result in one or multiple simultaneous intracerebral, subarachnoid, or lobar hemorrhages. Clinical dementia is seen in 10% to 30% of patients with CAA. Pathologically, 50%

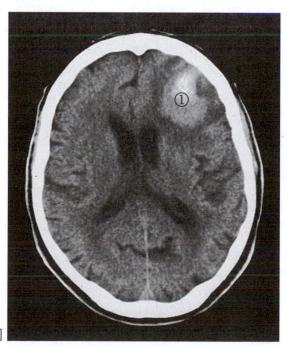

[A]

9 CVA DUE TO AMYLOID ANGIOPATHY

present with neuritic plaques. The characteristic lesion is **Congored-positive, apple-green, birefringent** amyloid in the media and adventitia of arteries.

Epidemiology   **Incidence increases with age**; seen in 60% of autopsies in those older than 90 years.

Management   IV **beta-blockers** to keep systolic BP < 150.

Complications   Recurrent stroke.

MINICASE 236: CAUDA EQUINA SYNDROME

A lesion affecting the nerve roots that branch off the end of the spinal cord (CAUDA EQUINA)
- caused by disk herniation, tumor, paraspinal abscess, or hematoma
- presents with low back pain, lower extremity sensory loss with sacral sparing, weakness, urinary and bowel incontinence, impotence, and loss of reflexes
- CT or MR demonstrates the lesion
- treatment is emergent surgical decompression for disk herniation, radiotherapy and surgery for tumor, and antibiotics and incision and drainage for abscess

---

MINICASE 237: CAVERNOUS SINUS THROMBOSIS

Thrombosis of the cavernous sinus and inflammation of its surrounding anatomic structures, including cranial nerves III, IV, V (ophthalmic and maxillary branches), and VI and the internal carotid artery
- classically presents with ptosis, proptosis, chemosis, and cranial nerve palsies (III, IV, V, and VI)
- usually secondary to infections of the face or paranasal sinuses (most commonly the sphenoid sinus)
- labs reveal elevated WBC count, wound or blood culture reveals *Staphylococcus aureus*, MR demonstrates lack or irregular enhancement of cavernous sinus
- lumbar puncture necessary to rule out meningitis
- treat with aggressive IV antibiotics (nafcillin, cefotaxime, metronidazole)
- the role of steroid and anticoagulant therapy is controversial
- complications include persistent oculomotor weakness, blindness, hemiparesis, and pituitary insufficiency

ID/CC A 62-year-old right-handed male with a history of hypertension and tobacco use is **unable to speak**.

HPI The patient was well this morning, but during a meeting his speech became slow and then stopped altogether. He was **able to follow instructions** to get up and walk but needed help walking. He was brought to the ER by a colleague. The patient has a history of **hypercholesterolemia**.

PE VS: normal HR; hypertension (BP 185/95). PE: alert and **able to follow commands** but **unable to repeat commands; nonfluent speech**; able to name two of three objects but unable to name parts of objects; right facial droop; right upper extremity 3/5, and right lower extremity 4/5 on motor exam.

Labs CBC/Lytes: normal. PT/PTT and glucose normal. ECG: sinus rhythm with LVH.

Imaging CT, brain (on admission): no hemorrhage; no mass; no shift. CT, brain (24 hours later): ischemic **infarct of the left posterior inferior frontal gyrus** (BROCA'S AREA). US, carotid: 80% left **ICA stenosis**. Echo: no thrombus.

Pathogenesis Broca's aphasia is a nonfluent (motor) aphasia characterized by broken speech in which patients are unable to produce spoken language, but **comprehension** of speech **remains intact**. Characteristically, patients are aware of their deficit and are frustrated with their inability to communicate. Hypertension, **diabetes**, cardiac disease, AIDS, drug abuse, heavy alcohol consumption, elevated serum cholesterol, and tobacco use are independent risk factors for the development of ischemic stroke.

Epidemiology An estimated 500,000 new cases of stroke of all types occur each year; strokes are a common cause of death and disability. Modifiable risk factors include tobacco use, hypertension, diabetes mellitus, and hypercholesterolemia.

Management **Antiplatelet agent** (e.g., aspirin) for secondary stroke prevention; heparin for DVT prophylaxis. Hold antihypertensive agents for 2 to 4 weeks, as cerebral hypoperfusion is a risk. Six weeks after stroke, obtain an MR to confirm the extent of ICA stenosis. **Carotid endarterectomy** is indicated if stenosis on symptomatic side is > 70%. Endarterectomy is not indicated until 6 weeks after acute stroke.

Complications Recurrent ischemic infarcts and CAD.

CVA, BROCA'S APHASIA

ID/CC A 57-year-old left-handed man complains of acute-onset, **severe headache** and then develops **weakness on the left side of his body** (HEMIPLEGIA).

HPI The patient has **hypertension** that has been treated with multiple antihypertensives. Three months ago, he stopped taking all his prescription medications (NONCOMPLIANT WITH MEDICATIONS). He was asymptomatic until this morning.

PE VS: **hypertension** (BP 205/110); normal HR. PE: lethargic; responsive to voices but unable to follow commands; positive doll's eyes; left facial droop but able to raise eyebrows (UPPER MOTOR NEURON LEFT FACIAL PALSY); motor strength 0/5 in left upper and lower extremity; left Babinski's present.

Labs CBC/Lytes: normal. Glucose normal, PT/PTT and platelets normal. ECG: sinus rhythm with LVH.

Imaging [A] CT, head: focal hemorrhage involving the right basal ganglia.

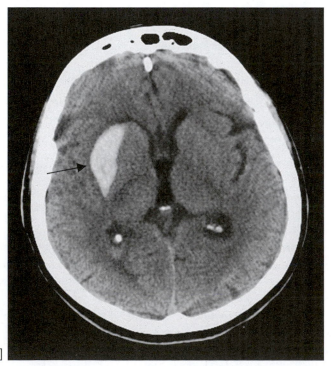

[A]

Pathogenesis	The **most common causes** of intracerebral hemorrhage are **hypertension, vascular malformation, tumor**, and **cerebral amyloid angiopathy**. The most common sites of hypertensive hemorrhage are the basal ganglia (putamen and thalamus), cerebellum, and pons.
Epidemiology	Fifteen percent of all strokes are hemorrhagic.
Management	**Intubate** for airway protection; administer **IV beta-blockers to keep systolic BP < 150** (try to reduce blood pressure to the lowest level that can maintain cerebral perfusion). Mechanical hyperventilation and IV mannitol can be used if there is an increase in ICP. These treatments will provide time for surgical intervention to prevent brainstem herniation.
Complications	Complications include **recurrent stroke** and hypertensive encephalopathy. Early mortality rate is higher than observed in infarction. Level of consciousness is a strong prognostic factor. Comatose patients have a mortality rate of approximately 90%.

MINICASE 238: CEREBELLOPONTINE ANGLE COMPRESSION

An acoustic neuroma, meningioma, metastatic lesion, or cholesteatoma compressing the cerebellopontine angle
• presents with unilateral hearing loss, tinnitus, vertigo, and facial nerve palsy
• CT or MR demonstrates mass lesion
• treat with radiation therapy to shrink the tumor or surgical resection
• complications include increased ICP

MINICASE 239: CEREBRAL ANEURYSM

Outpouchings on arteries caused by a combination of congenital defects in the vascular wall and degenerative changes, usually occurring at branching sites on the large arteries of the circle of Willis at the base of the brain
• rupture usually presents with sudden severe headache, vomiting, and increased intracranial pressure
• noncontrast CT scan demonstrates clot in the subarachnoid space
• treat acutely with short-acting analgesics, sedation, intubation as necessary
• institute anticonvulsant (phenytoin) and vasospasm prophylaxis (nimodipine), definitively manage with endovascular therapy or surgical clipping of aneurysm
• complications include rebleeding, vasospasm, hydrocephalus, SIADH, and seizures

ID/CC   A 74-year-old African-American male with a history of **hypertension** and **non-insulin-dependent diabetes mellitus** (NIDDM) complains of sudden-onset **weakness in his right hand** and **drooling**.

HPI   He was asymptomatic when he went to bed, but when he woke up he noted clumsiness while brushing his teeth. He also noted drooling out of the right side of his mouth.

PE   VS: **hypertension** (BP 175/95). PE: alert and oriented; dysarthric; right facial droop with no forehead weakness (due to UMN right facial nerve palsy); motor strength 4/5 in right arm, 5/5 in right leg, and 5/5 in left arm and leg; reflexes 2+ and symmetric; Babinski's absent; sensory exam normal.

Labs   CBC: normal. Blood glucose elevated; **hypercholesterolemia** (LDL 295 mg/dL). ECG: sinus rhythm with LVH.

Imaging   CT, brain (on admission): no mass; no shift; no hemorrhage; periventricular white matter disease consistent with small-vessel ischemia. CT, head (24 hours after admission): lacunar ischemic infarct in the posterior limb of the left internal capsule (due to involvement of thalamoperforate arteries). **[A]** CT, head: a

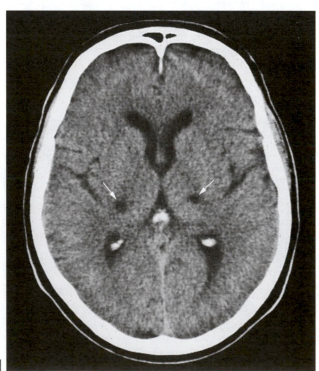

[A]

CVA, LACUNAR STROKE

different case showing bilateral lacunar infarcts. US, carotid: no significant stenosis. Echo: no thrombus; LVH.

Pathogenesis Lacunar infarcts are caused by occlusion of penetrating branches of the circle of Willis, MCA, or vertebral and basilar arteries due to thrombosis or lipohyalinotic thickening of these branches.

Epidemiology Lacunar strokes account for approximately 20% of all strokes.

Management **Antiplatelet agents** (e.g., aspirin, ticlopidine) reduce stroke risk by 25%; begin after the initial head CT has ruled out cerebral hemorrhage. **Heparin** is given for DVT prophylaxis, and **lipid-lowering drugs** are given to reduce the risk of further strokes. Physical and occupational therapy are often useful in achieving maximal function.

Complications Lacunar stroke patients have a 15% chance of recurrence after initial recovery, with an 8% mortality rate.

MINICASE 240: CONUS MEDULLARIS LESION

A lesion of the terminal portion of the spinal cord (CONUS MEDULLARIS), usually between L1 and L2, caused by compression from disk herniation, tumor, paraspinal abscess, or hematoma
- presents with saddle anesthesia, impotence, and incontinence
- CT or MR demonstrates cord lesion
- treatment is surgical decompression for disk herniation, surgery with radiotherapy for tumor, and antibiotics and incision and drainage for abscess

MINICASE 241: CORD COMPRESSION—EXTRADURAL

Spinal cord impingement by a rapidly growing metastatic tumor, paraspinal abscess, disk herniation, or epidural hematoma
- presents with rapid-onset back pain, dermatomal sensory loss, paresis or paralysis, hyperreflexia, and incontinence
- CT or MR demonstrates spinal cord compression
- treatment is urgent decompression with radiation therapy, surgical excision, or antibiotics and incision and drainage (for treatment of an epidural abscess)

ID/CC A 91-year-old right-handed woman is found on the floor **unable to speak or move the right side of her body**.

HPI The patient lives alone and was last seen 2 days ago. The woman was grunting and not moving her right side.

PE VS: **hypotension** (BP 80/50); **irregularly irregular pulse** (due to atrial fibrillation; average HR 110). PE: alert; unable to speak spontaneously or to repeat or follow commands; motor strength 0/5 in right arm and leg with Babinski's present; reflexes 2+ and symmetric; no cranial nerve palsies.

Labs CBC normal. Elevated BUN (55 mg/dL); normal creatinine (1.1 mg/dL) (prerenal azotemia due to dehydration or low cardiac output). Lytes: normal. ECG: **atrial fibrillation** with fast ventricular rate.

Imaging [A] CT, head: hypodensity (1) involving the entire left MCA distribution (classic sign of completed ischemic infarct). Echo: no thrombus; dilated left atrium; LV ejection fraction of 55%.

Pathogenesis Left MCA occlusion causes **contralateral hemiplegia, hemisensory loss**, and **loss of right visual field** (HOMONYMOUS

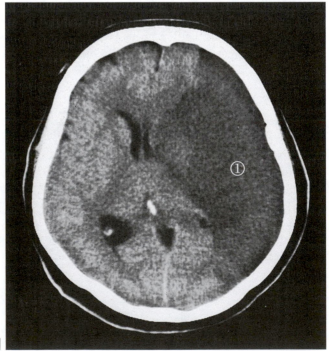

[A]

HEMIANOPSIA). The inability to speak, repeat, and understand language (GLOBAL APHASIA) results when the dominant hemisphere is involved, including Broca's area, Wernicke's area, and the arcuate fasciculus.

Epidemiology   The annual risk of stroke with atrial fibrillation is 5%.

Management   Prevent recurrent strokes in those with atrial fibrillation by placing on **long-term anticoagulation with warfarin**. For maximal recovery after this event, physical, occupational, and speech therapy are necessary.

Complications   The most common complications are pneumonia and UTI due to Foley catheterization. Other complications include hemorrhagic transformation of the ischemic infarct and recurrent infarcts. Left MCA infarction also causes aphasia, alexia, agraphia, acalculia, and right/left confusion in addition to right-sided hemiplegia.

MINICASE 242: CORD COMPRESSION—INTRADURAL

Spinal cord impingement by a slow-growing primary malignancy, commonly a meningioma, hemangioblastoma, or astrocytoma
- presents with subacute back pain, dermatomal paresis, loss of sensation, and diminished reflexes
- CT or MR demonstrates spinal cord compression
- treatment is radiotherapy or surgical excision of the compressing lesion

---

MINICASE 243: EATON–LAMBERT SYNDROME

A paraneoplastic myasthenia-like syndrome due to antibodies directed at presynaptic calcium ion channels at the neuromuscular junction
- presents with weakness (usually proximal) and autonomic dysfunction
- EMG shows diagnostic increase in action potential with repetitive stimulation
- treat with corticosteroids or plasmapheresis, treat the underlying carcinoma

---

ID/CC A 55-year-old right-handed female with **chronic hypertension** presents with **acute-onset left-sided weakness** and **altered sensorium**.

HPI The patient is being treated for hypertension. This morning, her husband found her on the floor next to the bed unable to move her left arm and leg. She could speak but was "acting funny."

PE VS: **hypertension** (BP 180/100). PE: alert with fluent speech; answers questions appropriately but is **unable to draw a clock or copy a five-sided figure correctly; eyes deviated to right**; sensation absent to pinprick in left arm and leg; **0/5 strength in left arm and leg** and 5/5 strength in right arm and leg; DTRs 2+ in right arm and leg and 3+ in left arm and leg; increased tone in left arm and leg, normal in right arm and leg; Babinski's present on left; no carotid or subclavian bruit; no cardiac murmurs.

Labs CBC/Lytes: normal. PT/PTT and glucose normal. VDRL negative; antiphospholipid antibodies negative; elevated cholesterol and triglycerides.

Imaging CT, head (within 24 hours): no mass, hemorrhage, or midline shift. **[A]** CT, head (after 48 hours): right MCA infarct with extensive hypodensity (1). **[B]** MR, brain: another patient with a smaller T2-hyperintense right MCA infarct.

Pathogenesis Hypertension is an independent risk factor for the development of ischemic stroke. Right MCA occlusion causes **contralateral hemiplegia, hemisensory loss**, spatial agnosia, and **loss of left visual field** (HOMONYMOUS HEMIANOPIA) with **deviation of the eyes to the side of the lesion**. There is also global aphasia if the dominant hemisphere is affected.

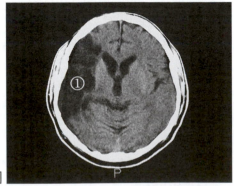
[A]

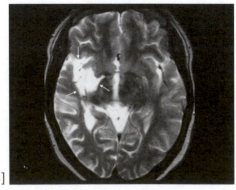
[B]

Epidemiology	There are 500,000 new strokes each year in the United States. Strokes are a common cause of disability. Modifiable risk factors include **tobacco use, hypertension, diabetes mellitus**, and **hypercholesterolemia**.
Management	**Avoid a precipitous fall in blood pressure** in order to maintain adequate cerebral perfusion. **Antiplatelet agents** reduce stroke risk by 25%; begin them after the initial head CT has ruled out cerebral hemorrhage. **Lipid-lowering drugs** also reduce the risk of recurrent stroke.
Complications	Complications include recurrent stroke, MI, DVT, UTI, and aspiration pneumonia. Loss of consciousness renders a poorer prognosis.

MINICASE 244: FETAL ALCOHOL SYNDROME

The leading cause of fetal malformations in the United States
- presents with microcephaly, growth retardation, and mental retardation
- CXR reveals cardiomegaly
- no specific treatment
- complications include cardiac septal defects

MINICASE 245: GERSTMANN–STRÄUSSLER–SCHEINKER SYNDROME

Rare spinocerebellar degeneration
- hereditary, with an onset in mid-adulthood
- presents with progressive ataxia, nystagmus, and extrapyramidal signs
- there is no proven treatment

MINICASE 246: KLUMPKE'S PALSY

Abduction injury affecting the lower brachial plexus (C7, C8, and T1 roots), producing paralysis of the muscles innervated by them
- causes include shoulder dystocia during birth
- presents with hand in "claw position" (due to paralysis of the ulnar nerve) and Horner's syndrome (due to damage to the sympathetic fibers of C8 and T1)
- treat with physiotherapy or nerve repair

ID/CC A 42-year-old **woman** presents with impaired consciousness and **left facial droop**.

HPI According to a witness, she complained of the acute onset of a severe, **"worst-ever" headache** followed by nausea and vomiting. Shortly thereafter she had a seizure and was then stuporous.

PE VS: tachycardia (HR 112); slight fever (37.8°C). PE: moaning, irritable, and confused; depressed level of consciousness; **nuchal rigidity; Kernig's and Brudzinski's signs positive; left facial droop; left hemiplegia; left hyperreflexia**; funduscopy reveals **papilledema**.

Labs CBC: normal. Lytes: hyponatremia (due to SIADH). PT/PTT normal (rules out SAH due to blood dyscrasias). ECG: inverted T waves (ROLLER COASTER T WAVES). LP: not done, since CT provides clear evidence of SAH and evidence of increased intracranial pressure from funduscopic exam.

Imaging **[A]** CT, head: hyperdensity (1) in the right MCA region representing hemorrhage from a ruptured aneurysm, with bilateral hyperdensities in sulci consistent with SAH. **[B]** CT, head: another SAH with the circle of Willis outlined by hyperdense subarachnoid blood.

Pathogenesis The most common cause of spontaneous SAH is **ruptured berry aneurysm**. Aneurysms (which can be seen in an angiogram **[C]**) develop because of a congenital weakness at **points of bifurcation in the circle of Willis**.

Epidemiology Shows slight female predominance.

Management Seizure prophylaxis with phenytoin and the calcium channel blocker **nimodipine** to prevent vasospasm. Obtain a **cerebral angiogram** of all four vessels as soon as possible. **Surgical aneurysm repair** should be performed within 48 hours to ensure maximal recovery. Patients with serious neurologic deficits do not benefit from early surgery. Aneurysms > 7 mm require prophylactic surgery. If present, hydrocephalus requires ventriculostomy or ventriculoperitoneal shunting.

Complications **Vasospasm** (most common cause of death) leads to infarction of surrounding tissue; blood in the subarachnoid space or cerebral cortex acts as a **seizure** focus. Other complications include cranial nerve palsies (most commonly CN III), **hydrocephalus,**

high-protein pulmonary edema, rebleed, and severe hyponatremia due to **SIADH**.

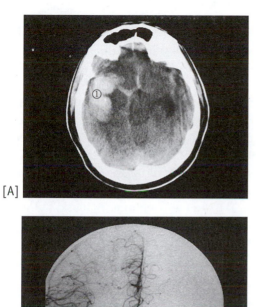

[A]

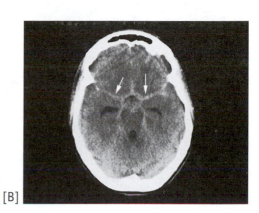

[B]

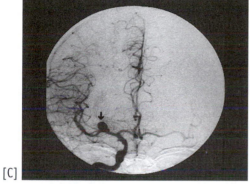

[C]

ID/CC	A 62-year-old right-handed female with a history of **paroxysmal atrial tachycardia** is brought to the hospital after "not making sense" at work.
HPI	The patient was at a meeting when she suddenly began **speaking "gibberish."** She was **unable to follow instructions** to get up. However, once her colleague helped her up, she was able to walk to the car without assistance.
PE	VS: **hypertension** (BP 160/100); **pulse irregularly irregular**. PE: alert and in no acute distress with clear but unintelligible speech (FLUENT APHASIA); **unable to repeat phrases** or follow commands; **paraphasic errors** (e.g., "shoon" instead of "spoon") and **neologisms** (nonexistent words, e.g., "bork"); cranial nerves intact; motor strength 5/5 and DTRs 2+ throughout; Babinski's absent.
Labs	CBC: normal. ECG: atrial fibrillation with controlled ventricular rate. Lytes: normal. PT/PTT and glucose normal.
Imaging	CT, head (on admission): no mass; no hemorrhage; no infarct. CT, head (24 hours after admission): ischemic infarct in the left superior temporal gyrus. US, carotid: no hemodynamically significant stenosis. Echo: dilated left atrium; no thrombus.
Pathogenesis	Wernicke's aphasia is typically due to a **cardioembolic event**. Patients are often unaware that their speech is incomprehensible.
Epidemiology	The annual risk of stroke with atrial fibrillation is 5%.
Management	To prevent recurrent strokes, patients with atrial fibrillation should be placed on **lifelong anticoagulation** with **warfarin** and/or **antiplatelet** agents. Speech therapy is useful.
Complications	Recurrent stroke and MI.

CVA, WERNICKE'S APHASIA

ID/CC   An **81-year-old** right-handed **male** with a history of insulin-dependent diabetes mellitus (IDDM) and **hypertension** presents with gradually progressing confusion over the past several years.

HPI   He has had **two strokes** with residual left hemiparesis; he was brought to the hospital by his wife due to **increasing confusion** and **angry outbursts**. He has forgotten important appointments, repeatedly **asks the same questions**, and **forgets names** (all due to memory impairment). He has also become irritable, easily frustrated, and suspicious and demanding of his wife (all due to behavioral impairment). For the past 2 years he has not driven a car because he becomes confused at intersections. He has recently been **getting lost** when he takes walks (due to visual and spatial disorientation).

PE   VS: **hypertension** (BP 150/90). PE: pleasant and alert; **oriented to person only**; speech fluent; **cannot recall current president or recent news events**, and **cannot perform mathematical calculations** (serial sevens, simple addition and subtraction); mild left facial droop; 4/5 strength in left upper and lower extremities with mild increase in tone; 5/5 strength in right upper and lower extremities; DTRs 3+ in left upper and lower extremities and 2+ in right upper and lower extremities; **positive snout and palmar-mental reflexes** (PRIMITIVE REFLEXES); **Babinski's present bilaterally** (sign of global hemispheric dysfunction); withdraws to pain in all four extremities; finger-to-nose intact bilaterally.

Labs   CBC: normal. Serum VDRL, TFTs, B_{12}, and folate levels normal. EEG: moderate to marked generalized slowing; no epileptiform activity.

Imaging   CT, head: diffuse **periventricular hypodensity**; small old ischemic infarcts; no hemorrhage; no mass.

Pathogenesis   Vascular dementia is an accumulation of defects from **multiple, bilateral cerebral infarcts**. Patients with previous cerebral insults will have reduced cerebral reserve and are more vulnerable to confusion from minor insults. Dementia can be classified as cortical or subcortical. **Cortical** causes include primary degenerative dementias such as Alzheimer's, Pick's disease, Creutzfeldt-Jakob disease, multi-infarct dementia, and dementias due to other causes such as normal pressure hydrocephalus, mass lesions, drugs, and HIV. **Subcortical** dementias include Parkinson's and Huntington's dementia.

DEMENTIA—VASCULAR

Epidemiology	Causes 15% to 30% of all dementias; typically occurs in **patients older than 50 years** with a **history of generalized atherosclerotic disease. Men** are affected more often than women.
Management	Aggressive **control of hypertension**, hyperlipidemia, and diabetes to prevent further decline. Medium-potency **neuroleptics** such as thioridazine may be administered for control of aggressive behavior.
Complications	Urinary incontinence, seizure disorder (infarcted regions can serve as a seizure focus), and dysphagia resulting in aspiration pneumonia.

MINICASE 247: LUMBAR SPINAL STENOSIS

May mimic cord compression
- usually due to congenital narrowing of the spinal canal exacerbated by degenerative osteoarthritic changes or hypertrophy of the facet joints, causing pressure on nerve roots
- presents with pseudoclaudication (pain in the leg or back occurring during walking) relieved by sitting forward
- CT/MR demonstrate spinal canal narrowing
- treat with surgical decompression (laminectomy)

MINICASE 248: MALIGNANT HYPERTHERMIA

A lethal, genetic myopathy triggered by inhalation anesthetics such as halothane, particularly if coupled with succinylcholine
- presents with fever, tachycardia, hypertension, acidosis, hyperkalemia, and muscle rigidity
- treat with cooling measures, dantrolene, IV fluids

MINICASE 249: MENINGIOMA

The most common benign extra-axial CNS tumor in adults
- presents with focal neurologic deficits, vision changes, headache, nausea, and vomiting
- MR or CT demonstrates mass lesion
- histology demonstrates whorled appearance and psammoma bodies
- treat with surgical resection
- excellent prognosis

Atlas Links: UCVI PG-P3-020, PM-P3-020

ID/CC	A **10-year-old** male is seen by a neurologist because of **progressive difficulty walking** and **diminution of vision**.
HPI	The patient has a **right foot deformity** (pes cavus). After suffering two episodes of syncope, he presented to a cardiologist and was diagnosed with **hypertrophic cardiomyopathy**. His parents give a history of **consanguineous marriage; an uncle**, who had a similar illness, **died of cardiac complications**.
PE	VS: normal. PE: wide-based **ataxia**; nystagmus; dysarthria; **areflexia** in lower extremities; **Babinski's present; joint position sense** and vibratory sense **lost in lower limbs**; pain and temperature sensations intact; intellect normal; spastic weakness in lower extremities with 4+ strength in select muscle groups in upper extremities; optic atrophy.
Labs	Elevated blood glucose (200 mg/dL; indicative of overt **diabetes mellitus**).
Pathogenesis	Friedreich's ataxia exhibits an **autosomal-recessive inheritance**; the gene locus has been mapped to chromosome 9. Classically, **three long tracts degenerate**: the pyramidal, dorsal, and spinocerebellar. Accompanying abnormalities include **cardiomyopathy**, skeletal abnormalities, optic atrophy, and an increased incidence of diabetes mellitus.
Epidemiology	Presents in children and involves ataxia with progressive involvement of all the extremities. The mean age of death is 31.
Management	No specific treatment is available.
Complications	**Cardiomyopathy is often the cause of death**, usually before age 40. Progressive neurologic decompensation results in loss of ambulation within 5 years after the onset of symptoms.

FRIEDREICH'S ATAXIA

ID/CC A **78-year-old** male nursing-home resident suffers a **generalized seizure**.

HPI The patient has never had a seizure before. He has experienced **headaches** that are worse in the morning and admits to occasional **nausea and vomiting**.

PE VS: **hypertension** (BP 150/90). PE: exhibits confusion; neck supple; **bilateral papilledema; Babinski's present on right side**; normal lung and skin exam.

Labs CBC: normal.

Imaging **[A]** CT, head: single, irregular enhancing left temporoparietal mass lesion with necrotic center (1), mass effect (2), and moderate surrounding edema.

Pathogenesis Glioblastoma multiforme is a **grade 4 astrocytoma** and is **markedly anaplastic**. Almost 75% of adult brain tumors are **supratentorial**, and the rest are in the posterior fossa. Histopathology reveals abundant necrosis. Metastases are uncommon.

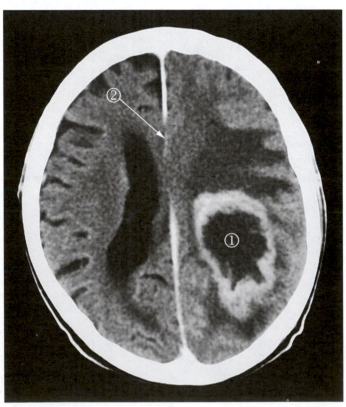

[A]

GLIOBLASTOMA MULTIFORME

Epidemiology	Occurs more commonly in **elderly individuals**, with a peak incidence in the seventh decade.
Management	**Tumor staging** is performed with CSF analysis, MRI, and angiography; **dexamethasone** is given to decrease brain edema; **phenytoin** is given as an anticonvulsant. Surgical resection is planned depending on the location and extent of the tumor. Radiation and chemotherapy usually follow. Usually fatal.
Complications	Hydrocephalus, seizures, herniation, and functional loss.
Atlas Links	ⓊⒸⓋⓉ PG-P3-012, PM-P3-012

MINICASE 250: MENINGITIS—LISTERIA

Caused by *Listeria monocytogenes*
- acquired in utero or through contaminated milk in neonates, or in debilitated adults (e.g., alcoholics, immunosuppressed)
- presents with high fever, headache, convulsions, and nuchal rigidity
- neutrophilic leukocytosis
- culture shows gram-positive bacillus
- treat with IV ampicillin, may combine with an aminoglycoside

Atlas Link: ⓊⒸⓋⓉ PG-M2-079

MINICASE 251: MENINGITIS—TUBERCULAR

Dissemination of primary TB to involve the meninges
- HIV increases risk
- presents with subacute headache, nuchal rigidity, communicating hydrocephalus, and cranial nerve palsies
- acid-fast bacilli in CSF
- cultures grow *Mycobacterium tuberculosis*
- treat with anti-TB drugs, corticosteroids if cerebral edema
- often leaves permanent neurologic changes

MINICASE 252: METASTATIC BRAIN TUMOR

Commonly caused by lung, breast, melanoma, kidney, and GI metastases
- presents with acute-onset focal neurologic deficits, headache, nausea, vomiting, and altered mental status
- MR and CT show small, well-circumscribed lesions at white-gray junction
- treat with local irradiation, treat underlying malignancy

Atlas Link: ⓊⒸⓋⓉ PM-P3-021

ID/CC	A 33-year-old woman who **recently had a URI** now complains of **loss of strength in her lower legs** and difficulty walking.
HPI	Over the past 4 weeks, she has noted **symmetric weakness** starting in her lower limbs and progressing to her hips and upper limbs (ASCENDING PARALYSIS). Over the past week she has experienced occasional urinary incontinence, lightheadedness on rising quickly, and shortness of breath.
PE	VS: no fever; **orthostatic hypotension; tachycardia** (due to autonomic dysfunction). PE: mental status normal; marked symmetric **loss of motor strength** with **flaccidity** most notable in **proximal lower limbs; absent patellar and Achilles reflexes bilaterally**; mild facial weakness.
Labs	LP: **elevated protein in CSF; normal cellularity** (CYTOALBUMINIC DISSOCIATION). Serum B_{12} normal; FTA negative; glucose normal. Lytes: normal. EMG: markedly slowed motor and sensory conduction. Nerve conduction studies reveal evidence of **demyelination** with **slowing of conduction velocity** and multifocal conduction blocks.
Imaging	CT/MR, brain: no intracranial lesions or hemorrhage.
Pathogenesis	Guillain–Barré syndrome is an acute demyelinating polyradiculoneuropathy that is believed to be an **autoimmune-mediated reaction** to certain infectious agents. The most common pathogens are thought to be *Campylobacter jejuni*, viral hepatitis, and EBV. Guillain–Barré syndrome can also occur following influenza vaccinations.
Epidemiology	There is a bimodal age distribution, with most cases occurring in early adulthood or between 45 and 64 years. There is no known HLA association.
Management	**Plasmapheresis** is the treatment of choice. Patients with hemodynamic instability and children may be given **IV immunoglobulin**. Hospitalization for potential respiratory failure (and subsequent mechanical ventilation).
Complications	Can lead to **respiratory insufficiency** that may require ventilatory support. Approximately 85% of patients make a complete or nearly complete recovery, with the mortality rate standing at 3% to 4%. Mortality arises from cardiac arrhythmias or superimposed viral or bacterial pneumonia.

GUILLAIN–BARRÉ SYNDROME

ID/CC   A 30-year-old male complains of moderate **headache**, nausea, **vomiting, fever** with chills, and muscle aches for the past 2 days.

HPI   Three days ago, the patient's wife noted that he **started to "forget things."** He has also been unable to name familiar objects such as a radio. His wife has noted **speech difficulty** and episodes of irritable behavior over the past 24 hours. He has also been **smelling nonexistent odors** (olfactory hallucinations are common in HSV encephalitis).

PE   VS: **fever** (38.4°C); **tachycardia** (HR 120); **tachypnea** (RR 24). PE: mildly confused and disoriented; **mild nuchal rigidity**; speech notable for **paraphasic errors** (e.g., "shoon" instead of "spoon"); patient follows simple (one-step) commands and approximately 50% of complex (three-step) commands; he can draw a clock and bisect lines correctly (tests of nondominant parietal lobe function) and can add and subtract two-digit numbers but cannot perform simple (one-digit) multiplication problems; cranial nerves intact; motor strength 5/5 bilaterally; DTRs 2+ and symmetric throughout; patient withdraws limbs to painful stimuli.

Labs   CBC/Lytes: normal. PT/PTT, BUN, and creatinine normal. LFTs: normal. LP: opening pressure of 100 mm water; **protein elevated** (100 mg/dL); **glucose normal**; elevated WBC count with **mononuclear pleocytosis; red cells present**; CSF culture negative (positive in HSV-2); **HSV DNA PCR** in CSF positive.

Imaging   [A] and [B] CT, brain: bilateral temporal lobe hypodensity (1). MR, brain: **T2 hyperintensity** involving the cortex and white matter in the **temporal lobes**.

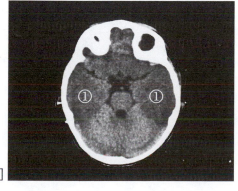
[A]

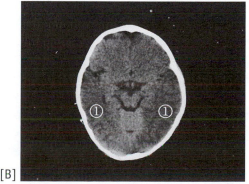
[B]

HERPES SIMPLEX ENCEPHALITIS

Pathogenesis   Ninety-five percent of cases of herpes simplex encephalitis are due to **HSV type 1**. The ports of entry are the oropharyngeal mucosa, conjunctiva, or broken skin; the virus **replicates locally and enters the sensory nerves**. From the sensory nerves, the virus is transported to the sensory nerve ganglia, where it remains latent. The factors that induce activation of the latent virus and the mechanism by which the virus targets the temporal lobes are not well understood.

Epidemiology   HSV encephalitis is the most common identified cause of acute sporadic viral encephalitis. HSV-1 encephalitis occurs in all age groups, in both sexes, and during all seasons.

Management   Untreated patients rapidly deteriorate to coma and death in 70% of cases. Treat with **IV acyclovir**. Mannitol and corticosteroids are given to relieve cerebral edema, and phenytoin is used to treat seizures. Repeat lumbar puncture after treatment to ensure that there is no residual infection.

Complications   Complications include persistent seizures, recurrent lymphocytic meningitis, and neurologic deficits. Amnesia is a prominent residual symptom.

Atlas Link   U C V 1 M-M2-089

MINICASE 253: MONONEURITIS MULTIPLEX

A broad term describing a pattern of nerve dysfunction in which affected nerves are individually identifiable
- common causes include polyarteritis nodosa, diabetes mellitus, rheumatoid arthritis, amyloidosis, HIV infection, and leprosy
- presents with diffuse involvement of both motor and sensory peripheral nerves
- nerve conduction studies demonstrate axonal damage
- treat the underlying disease

ID/CC	A 52-year-old male presents with **left eyelid droop** (PTOSIS) and **lack of perspiration** on the left side (ANHIDROSIS) following a motor vehicle accident.
HPI	The patient has no significant medical history. His car was rear-ended at a traffic light.
PE	VS: normal. PE: **left pupil constricted** (MIOSIS); left eyelid drooping; perspiration palpable on right side of forehead but not on left.
Labs	CBC: normal. PT/PTT: normal.
Imaging	US, carotid: occlusion of the left internal carotid artery consistent with carotid dissection.
Pathogenesis	The course of the **sympathetic tract** can be disrupted at a number of sites, causing Horner's syndrome. The syndrome may be caused by any lesion that disrupts the sympathetic fibers in the carotid plexus, cervical sympathetic chain, upper thoracic cord (e.g., superior sulcus or Pancoast's lung tumors), or brainstem (Wallenberg's syndrome).
Epidemiology	The syndrome is relatively rare.
Management	Manage these patients in the **ICU**. When the cause of Horner's is carotid dissection, IV **heparin** and 3 to 6 months of **warfarin** is the accepted treatment. Prevention of unequal pupils is impossible.

MINICASE 254: NARCOLEPSY

Sudden transition from state of consciousness directly into REM sleep
- strong genetic component (almost all cases are associated with HLA-DR15)
- presents with excessive daytime somnolence, hypnagogic (sleep-onset) hallucinations, cataplexy (sudden loss of muscle tone without loss of consciousness and elicited by emotion), and sleep paralysis (temporary paralysis of voluntary muscles on awakening)
- REM latency is markedly shortened (< 10 minutes)
- treat with methylphenidate to prevent daytime sleep, imipramine if significant cataplexy or hypnagogic hallucinations are present

HORNER'S SYNDROME

ID/CC A **38-year-old** woman presents with a 1-year history of progressively worsening **abrupt, involuntary jerking movements** of the limbs (CHOREA), absentmindedness, and slurred speech.

HPI The patient's family first noted her inability to button clothes. Movements began with facial twitches and now are coarse, **purposeless, dancelike movements of the extremities** that disappear during sleep. Family members also complain that the patient is depressed, irritable, impulsive, and emotionally labile. For the past 6 months, she has displayed memory impairment. The patient's **mother died of "dementia"** at the age of 55, and her **brother was placed in a nursing home** at the age of 48.

PE VS: normal. PE: blunted affect; unable to follow complex (three-step) commands; **lack of verbal and perceptual skills; deficits in attention**, organization, and sequencing abilities (due to frontal system dysfunction); short-term memory defective; diminished muscle tone.

Labs **Trinucleotide repeat** in Huntington gene on chromosome 4p.

Imaging **[A]** CT, head: bilateral cerebral atrophy; rounding (due to caudate atrophy) and enlargement of the anterior horns of the lateral ventricles.

Pathogenesis An **autosomal-dominant** condition with **high penetrance** characterized by widespread loss of neurons in the neostriatum, Huntington's disease is a chronic, progressive neurodegenerative disorder. The function of the Huntington gene is unknown. Successive generations exhibit **lengthening of the trinucleotide (CAG) repeat** (GENETIC ANTICIPATION) and thus experience onset at progressively **younger ages**.

Epidemiology Symptoms usually begin between 35 and 45 years.

Management No treatment is available for the underlying neurologic disease. **Haloperidol**, perphenazine, or drugs that **block dopamine receptors** or **deplete brain monoamines** reduce choreiform movements. Tricyclic antidepressants or SSRIs for depression. Concurrent use of MAO inhibitors and tricyclic antidepressants is contraindicated.

HUNTINGTON'S DISEASE

Complications Patients may develop dysphagia and become progressively rigid and bedridden. Death is typically due to infections such as pneumonia or UTI.

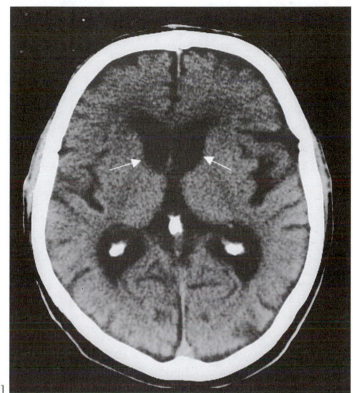

[A]

ID/CC	A **4-year-old boy** presents with **headache** and **awkward gait**.
HPI	His symptoms have been present for 3 months. His parents have noted that he "walks into the wall." Over the past week, he has **vomited** daily.
PE	VS: normal. PE: bilateral **papilledema**; strength 5/5 throughout; **ataxic gait**; neck supple.
Labs	CBC/Lytes: normal. PT/PTT: normal.
Imaging	**[A]** CT, head: **midline cerebellar mass** (1) with surrounding edema and enlarged ventricles. **[B]** CT, head (contrast): a different case with an enhancing cerebellar vermis mass (1) and obstructive hydrocephalus.
Pathogenesis	This highly malignant tumor arises from neural precursor cells on the **floor of the fourth ventricle** and may block the flow of CSF, resulting in increased ICP.
Epidemiology	Infratentorial medulloblastomas are the most common malignant brain tumor in children. The **male-to-female ratio is 2 to 1**; five-year survival is 50%.
Management	**Surgery** is performed to establish the diagnosis and debulk the tumor. Then **radiotherapy** and/or chemotherapy is initiated.
Complications	Radiotherapy may lead to cognitive delay as well as to endocrine abnormalities. **Metastasis** to meninges and spinal cord.
Atlas Link	UCV1 PG-P3-018

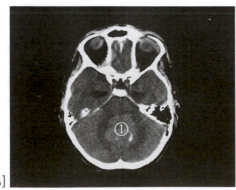

[A]

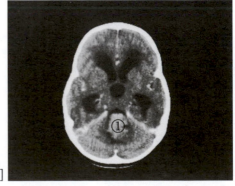

[B]

ID/CC   A **35-year-old** male complains of intermittent **episodes** of **nausea** and **dizziness** over the past month.

HPI   At first the patient had episodes of nausea and a sensation that the **"room was spinning"** (VERTIGO); these episodes lasted 3 to 5 minutes. Over the past week, however, the symptoms have persisted for 1 to 2 hours. A severe episode two days ago resulted in emesis and "buzzing" in the left ear (TINNITUS).

PE   VS: normal. PE: mild sensorineural hearing loss in left ear; **Bárány maneuver** fails to reproduce sensation of vertigo; remainder of neurologic exam normal.

Labs   CBC: normal. Serum VDRL negative.

Imaging   MR, brain: unremarkable.

Pathogenesis   Ménière's disease is caused by an **increase in volume of the endolymphatic system** (ENDOLYMPHATIC HYDROPS), resulting in distention. The primary lesion is thought to be in the endolymphatic sac, which is responsible for endolymph filtration and excretion. Two known causes are syphilis and head trauma.

Epidemiology   Typical onset is in middle age.

Management   Treat acute attacks with **bed rest; meclizine** or **dimenhydrinate** is used for symptomatic relief of vertigo. Chronic treatment involves institution of a **low-sodium diet** and **diuretics**. To treat intractable disease, a **surgical shunt** should be placed (relieves vertigo in 70% of cases but causes hearing loss in 50%).

Complications   **Remissions and relapses** may occur throughout life; gradual **hearing loss** due to multiple attacks is possible.

MÉNIÈRE'S DISEASE

ID/CC	A 25-year-old woman presents with **frontal headache**, fever, photophobia, and **neck stiffness** of 2 days' duration.
HPI	She had a URI 2 weeks ago. She now also complains of nausea and **vomiting**.
PE	VS: fever. PE: alert and oriented; **mild nuchal rigidity; Kernig's and Brudzinski's signs negative**; no focal deficits; funduscopy normal.
Labs	CBC: normal. Lytes: normal (serum glucose 125 mg/dL). LP: opening pressure 11 cm water; clear; CSF **glucose 100 mg/dL; 20 WBCs with 90% lymphocytes; mildly elevated protein**; CSF Gram stain reveals no organisms.
Imaging	CT, head: normal.
Pathogenesis	Meningitis is an inflammation of the leptomeninges and presents as CSF pleocytosis. Enteroviruses, mumps virus, arbovirus, HSV, HIV, and medications (ibuprofen) are causes of aseptic meningitis.
Epidemiology	Incidence is 1 in 10,000 per year. A specific pathogen is rarely identified.
Management	Treat with bed rest, analgesics, and antipyretics. Typically runs a benign, short (2- to 3-day) course.
Complications	The prognosis is excellent in adults; rare complications in infants include hearing loss and learning disabilities. Hyponatremia may develop as a result of SIADH.

MINICASE 255: NEUROFIBROMATOSIS TYPE 1

Also called von Recklinghausen's disease, a multisystem genetic disorder that is commonly associated with cutaneous, neurologic, and orthopedic manifestations resulting from a mutation in or deletion of the NF1 gene on chromosome 17
- presents with multiple café-au-lait spots, subcutaneous neurofibromas, optic nerve tumors, Lisch nodules (iris hamartomas), bone abnormalities, and pheochromocytomas
- symptomatic treatment
- complications include malignant transformation of neurofibromas, hypertension, and brain tumors (neurofibrosarcomas)

Atlas Links: ⬚⬚⬚⬚ MC-255A, MC-255B

MENINGITIS—ASEPTIC

ID/CC   A 50-year-old male presents with **high fever** with chills, severe **headache**, and a **declining mental status**.

HPI   The patient is homeless and had been complaining of cough and fever for the last week. He was found in a stupor.

PE   VS: fever (39.5°C); **tachycardia** (HR 130); tachypnea; hypotension (BP 90/60). PE: nonverbal, confused, disoriented, and unable to follow commands; no skin rashes (meningococcal meningitis less likely); nuchal rigidity; **Kernig's and Brudzinski's signs positive**; no cranial nerve palsies; Babinski's absent; funduscopy normal.

Labs   CBC: leukocytosis (20,000). Normal serum glucose (110 mg/dL). LP: **opening pressure 25 cm water; 2,000 WBCs/μL** (90% PMNs); **glucose 20 mg/dL; protein 170 mg/dL**; CSF Gram stain reveals **gram-positive cocci** in chains. Culture yields *Streptococcus pneumoniae*.

Imaging   CT, head: normal.

Pathogenesis   Bacteria may infiltrate the meninges via the blood or from adjacent structures; **hematogenous spread is most common** and typically occurs via the upper respiratory tract. Low glucose in the CSF, high protein, and marked pleocytosis are characteristic of bacterial meningitis; **Gram stain**, which is positive in 80% of cases, is diagnostic. The most common organisms involved are *Haemophilus influenzae*, *Neisseria meningitidis*, and *S. pneumoniae*.

Epidemiology   *S. pneumoniae* **is the most common cause of meningitis in adults** and the second most common cause in children older than 6 years.

Management   Empiric IV ceftriaxone and vancomycin; then narrow the antibiotic spectrum when organism susceptibility results return. In cases of increased ICP, **steroids** should be used.

Complications   Pneumococcal meningitis has a significant mortality rate and is associated with residual neurologic deficits, seizures, and sepsis. Coma and pneumonia are associated with a poor prognosis. Rapid killing of bacteria may result in inflammation that leads to increased permeability of the blood-brain barrier, edema, and increased ICP.

Atlas Links   [UCV1] M-M2-092, PG-M2-092A, PG-M2-092B

MENINGITIS—BACTERIAL

ID/CC	A **21-year-old female** presents with a history of **intermittent, severe headaches** of 3 years' duration.
HPI	The patient gets headaches approximately six times per year. The headaches begin with light flashes in the right visual field that last for 15 to 20 minutes; approximately 10 minutes later, a **unilateral** left **temporal throbbing pain** begins. The pain increases in severity and then lasts for 10 to 12 hours. Occasionally the headaches are **associated with nausea and vomiting**. In addition, the patient cannot bear light, movement, or noise. She has a **family history of migraine**.
PE	VS: stable. PE: funduscopy reveals sharp disks bilaterally; visual acuity 20/20 bilaterally; remainder of neurologic exam normal.
Labs	CBC/Lytes: normal. ESR: normal (check for temporal arteritis).
Pathogenesis	Individuals have noted various **precipitants** to migraines, including red wine, exercise, menstruation, estrogen, caffeine, lack of sleep, and skipping of meals. Migraine can occur with **aura** (a transient neurologic dysfunction, usually visual in nature, that occurs within 60 minutes before or after headache onset).
Epidemiology	Most commonly, the initial attack is during **teenage years**. More **common in females** after puberty.
Management	**Prophylaxis** with **beta-blockers, verapamil**, or **valproic acid. Abortive treatment** consists of **NSAIDs, sumatriptan**, and **dihydroergotamine nasal spray**.

MINICASE 256: OBSTRUCTIVE HYDROCEPHALUS

Results from obstruction to the flow of CSF (intraventricular or extraventricular), with most cases due to stenoses of the aqueduct of Sylvius, Arnold–Chiari malformation, mass lesion, or infection
- may also be idiopathic
- infants present with poor feeding, irritability, head enlargement, and "setting-sun" sign (both ocular globes are deviated downward)
- MR shows dilated lateral ventricles and dilated third ventricle
- treat by surgical insertion of shunt either from the lateral ventricle to the IVC or directly from the third ventricle to the subarachnoid space

ID/CC A **30-year-old woman** complains of gradual diminution of vision in the right eye.

HPI She has had several **prior neurologic symptoms**, including an episode of loss of sensation and tingling in her left leg 1 year ago that lasted 2 to 3 days; she did not seek medical attention at that time. She has noted a gradual decrease of vision in her right eye over the last week, with discomfort on moving the right eye.

PE VS: normal. PE: nystagmus; unable to adduct eyes on lateral gaze (internuclear ophthalmoplegia); swollen right optic nerve (due to optic neuritis) with blurred margins; visual acuity 20/400 in right eye and 20/20 in left eye; **DTRs asymmetrically hyperactive**; sensory and cerebellar exam intact; upon flexion of neck, she reports feeling "electric shocks" down her spine (LHERMITTE'S SIGN).

Labs LP: CSF shows **lymphocytic pleocytosis, oligoclonal bands** (most specific lab abnormality), elevated myelin basic protein, and negative Lyme titer. Impaired visual, auditory, and somatosensory evoked responses.

Imaging [A] MR, brain: **multiple periventricular white matter lesions** on T2-weighted image. [B] MR, spine: large hyperintense plaque of demyelination at C5 level.

Pathogenesis Multiple sclerosis (MS) is probably an autoimmune process triggered by a virus (via molecular mimicry) occurring in a genetically susceptible person. The specific pathology is **demyelination** with axonal sparing. Any area of the CNS may be involved, but lesions commonly occur in the **lateral ventricular margins** of the **fourth ventricle**.

Epidemiology Mean age of onset is 32 years, with a female-to-male ratio of 2 to 1; 25% of patients have a **family history**. Frequency rate **declines with increasing proximity to the equator**.

Management Seventy percent of cases remit spontaneously. **Beta-Interferon** may be given to prevent recurrences in patients with relapsing MS. **Corticosteroids** are used for the treatment of acute relapses. **Anticholinergics** are given for urinary frequency and urgency; baclofen is useful in treating spasticity. Nocturnal spasms can be relieved by diazepam, and diffuse dysesthetic pain responds to carbamazepine or gabapentin.

MULTIPLE SCLEROSIS

Complications As the disease progresses there is increased motor tone and spasticity, bladder dysfunction, and fatigue.

Atlas Link UCV1 PG-P3-023

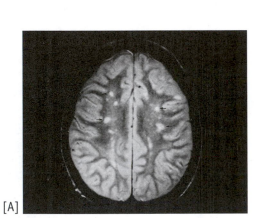

[A]

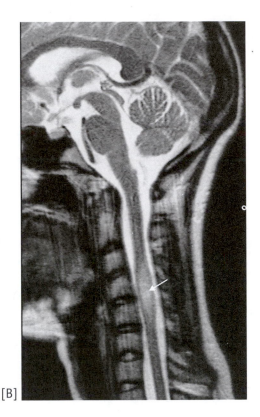

[B]

ID/CC A **40-year-old woman** complains of **occasional double vision** and "droopy" eyelids.

HPI For the past 3 months, she has noted intermittent diplopia that arises when she is watching television. Her husband adds that her **eyelids become droopy at night but are normal in the morning**.

PE VS: normal. PE: **bilateral ptosis** that **worsens with repeated blinking**; extraocular muscles intact, with diplopia on extremes of lateral gaze; motor strength 5/5 bilaterally on initial and 4/5 on prolonged testing; DTRs normal; sensory exam normal.

Labs **Elevated acetylcholine receptor antibody** titer. EMG: decrease in muscle action potential with repeated firing. **Tensilon** test (IV injection of acetylcholinesterase inhibitor) leads to resolution of ptosis and diplopia on lateral gaze.

Imaging **[A]** CT, chest: lobular **thymic mass** in the anterior mediastinum.

Pathogenesis Myasthenia gravis is an **autoimmune process**. Antibodies are produced to the acetylcholine receptor, resulting in the destruction of receptors and disruption of the neuromuscular

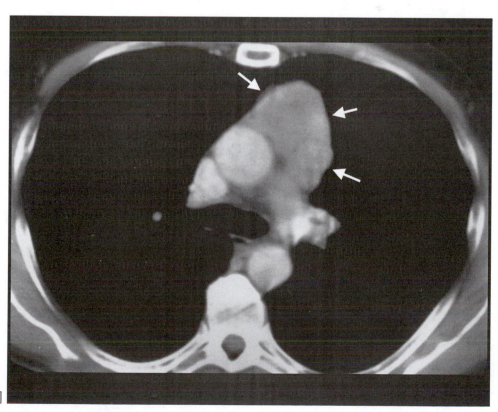

[A]

MYASTHENIA GRAVIS

junction. Can be distinguished clinically from Eaton–Lambert syndrome by **worsening rather than improving symptoms with repetitive motion**.

Epidemiology	Myasthenia gravis has a prevalence of approximately 1 in 7,000, with a peak incidence in younger women and older men.
Management	**Pyridostigmine**, a cholinesterase inhibitor, is used for symptomatic relief of weakness. Long-term **immunosuppression** with corticosteroids and azathioprine. Treat acute exacerbations with **plasmapheresis** and IV **immunoglobulin**. **Thymectomy** may help up to 85% of patients.
Complications	**Myasthenic crisis** is an acute exacerbation involving respiratory muscles that may require mechanical ventilation; it is often secondary to underlying infection.

MINICASE 257: OLIGODENDROGLIOMA

A slow-growing glial tumor that is relatively uncommon
- presents with focal neurologic findings, nausea, vomiting, and headache
- head CT shows a round, calcified, hypodense lesion
- treat with a combination of surgery, chemotherapy, and radiotherapy

---

MINICASE 258: OLIVOPONTOCEREBELLAR ATROPHY

Also known as spinocerebellar ataxia
- inherited as an autosomal-dominant trait
- presents with adult-onset cerebellar ataxia, dysarthria, and extrapyramidal signs
- there is no effective treatment

MINICASE 259: PERIPHERAL NEUROPATHY—DIABETIC

Insidious loss of peripheral or cranial nerve function related to chronic hyperglycemia
- presents with numbness, tingling, and burning in the lower extremities in a stocking-glove distribution
- EMG shows denervation
- treat with insulin for strict glycemic control (monitor with hemoglobin A1c levels), add carbamazepine for pain
- emphasize foot care to patients to prevent the development of ulcers

Atlas Link: ⊔©Ⅴ② MC-259

ID/CC   A 34-year-old male presents with **clumsiness of the hands** and multiple "falls."

HPI   The patient is an only child whose **mother died from a "heart attack"** at the age of 40. He has had increasing difficulty using tools, buttoning shirts, and tying his shoes. He has also begun to trip on the rugs at home. He has **difficulty releasing his grip** when shaking hands.

PE   VS: normal. PE: marked male-pattern **baldness; bilateral ptosis** with hollowing of masseter and temples (HATCHET FACE) and **bilateral facial weakness** (FISH MOUTH); testicular atrophy; percussion of thenar eminence produces abduction of thumb and firm contraction of thenar eminence (MYOTONIA); bilateral foot drop; weakness and difficulty relaxing distal muscles; sensory exam normal; DTRs reduced.

Labs   CBC: normal. Mildly elevated CK; **DNA analysis** reveals 100 copies of a **trinucleotide repeat in the myotonin gene**. EMG: **myotonic discharges**. Muscle biopsy reveals increased number of central nuclei, prominent ring fibers, and areas of disorganized sarcoplasm devoid of normal striations. ECG: **first-degree heart block**.

Pathogenesis   Myotonic dystrophy is inherited as an **autosomal-dominant** disorder. The defect consists of greater than 30 copies of a trinucleotide repeat in the myotonin gene; the function of the myotonin protein is, however, unknown. **Anticipation**, the phenomenon in which successive generations experience more severe disease, is due to expansion in the number of trinucleotide repeats from one generation to the next.

Epidemiology   Incidence is 13.5 in 100,000 live births. The most common muscular dystrophy seen among adults.

Management   Administer **phenytoin** or quinine to relieve myotonia. Use orthotic devices to alleviate foot drop. **Cardiac evaluation** should be performed owing to the high incidence of arrhythmias.

Complications   **Sudden death** due to cardiac conduction defects; cataracts; and testicular atrophy.

MYOTONIC DYSTROPHY

ID/CC	A **2-year-old girl** is brought to the ER by her parents, who have noticed a **bumpy right-sided abdominal mass**.
HPI	She is a healthy child who is up to date in her vaccinations. For the past week, her parents have noted the abdominal mass and occasional **diarrhea** (due to increased secretion of vasoactive intestinal peptide).
PE	VS: normal. PE: playful and in no acute distress; large right-sided abdominal mass with hard, irregular surface.
Labs	CBC: normal. UA: **elevated vanillylmandelic acid** (VMA is a catecholamine metabolite).
Imaging	MR, brain: normal. MR, spine: normal. CT, abdomen: **solid mass within the right adrenal gland** that enhances with contrast. CT, chest and pelvis: normal. Nuc: normal.
Pathogenesis	Neuroblastoma **arises from primitive neural crest cells** that form the adrenal medulla and the cervical and thoracic sympathetic chains. Approximately 70% of neuroblastomas **produce norepinephrine and its metabolites; 75% originate in the retroperitoneal area** and 55% originate in the adrenal gland. Poor prognosis is associated with *N-myc* overexpression, which is associated with a deletion of the short arm of chromosome 1.
Epidemiology	A common childhood tumor. Mean age of onset is 20 months. Two-thirds of cases occur within the **first 5 years of life**.
Management	Management consists of intensive surveillance of the entire body for metastases (spinal cord, retroperitoneal sympathetic ganglia, posterior mediastinum), **surgical resection** of any solid tumor (adrenal gland, brain), **chemotherapy** (vincristine, cyclophosphamide), and **radiotherapy**.
Complications	Complications include invasion of abdominal organs and **metastases** to **liver, lung**, and **bone**. Immunosuppression from chemotherapy and radiotherapy may cause subsequent **opportunistic infections**.
Atlas Links	[UCV1] PG-P3-026, PM-P3-026

ID/CC   A 72-year-old male presents with **memory loss, gait difficulty**, and **urinary incontinence**.

HPI   He was brought to the physician's office by his wife, who states that over the past year he has become increasingly forgetful. She adds that he has also wet his pants and their bed on several occasions (URINARY INCONTINENCE). For the past 6 months, the patient has fallen on numerous occasions and has had difficulty walking in his own home. He has a history of hypertension.

PE   VS: normal. PE: no speech defects; impaired short-term memory; unable to demonstrate how to comb his hair (impaired apraxia); motor strength 5/5 bilaterally throughout; DTRs 2+; gait characterized by short steps; patient can walk only 10 feet before having to sit down.

Labs   Serum B_{12}, folate, and TSH normal; VDRL negative. LP: **opening pressure of 90 mm H_2O**; normal glucose and protein; no nucleated cells. After 40 mL of CSF was removed, gait improved.

Imaging   **[A]** CT, head: **enlarged lateral ventricles** with comparatively normal sulci; periventricular white matter disease consistent with small-vessel ischemia; no mass, hemorrhage, cortical atrophy, or midline shift.

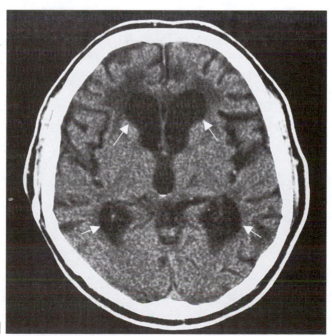

[A]

NORMAL PRESSURE HYDROCEPHALUS

Pathogenesis The etiology of normal pressure hydrocephalus is not known; it is likely due to decreased absorption of CSF across the arachnoid villi.

Management **Large-volume LP** often results in transient improvement. Approximately 30% to 50% of patients improve following placement of a **ventricular shunt**.

MINICASE 260: PROGRESSIVE MULTIFOCAL LEUKOENCEPHALOPATHY

Diffuse cerebral demyelination caused by JC virus in AIDS patients
• presents with diffuse neurologic dysfunction involving sensory and motor deficits
• MR shows large areas of demyelination bilaterally
• there is no treatment

MINICASE 261: PSEUDOBULBAR PALSY

A syndrome characterized by bulbar deficits
• etiologies include multi-infarct dementia and progressive supranuclear palsy
• presents with inappropriate, uncontrollable emotional outbursts (laughing, crying), dysarthria, dysphagia, and hyperactive gag and jaw-jerk reflexes
• treat the underlying hypertension to prevent new infarcts

MINICASE 262: SHY–DRAGER SYNDROME

Autonomic system failure, possibly related to degeneration of presympathetic neurons
• presents as orthostatic hypotension plus parkinsonism
• treat with fludrocortisone, salt tablets, and fluids to maintain intravascular volume
• consider an α-agonist (e.g., pseudoephedrine)

ID/CC	A **65-year-old** male complains of the development of a **hand tremor** coupled with **generalized muscle rigidity**.
HPI	His wife has noted generalized slowing of movement (BRADYKINESIA) and **lack of facial expression** (MASKLIKE FACIES) together with drooling. He has also noticed that his handwriting has been getting smaller (MICROGRAPHIA). The involuntary tremor decreases during voluntary motion.
PE	VS: normal. PE: severe seborrhea of scalp; sustained blinking follows tapping on nasal bridge (MYERSON'S SIGN); stooped posture; **postural instability; gait short- and slow-stepped** at first, followed by quick forward steps to prevent fall (FESTINANT GAIT), with no arm swing; intermittent muscle spasms with passive movement of joints (COGWHEEL RIGIDITY); DTRs normal; flexor plantar responses.
Labs	ESR: normal. Lytes/LFTs: normal. TSH: normal.
Imaging	CXR/KUB: within normal limits.
Pathogenesis	Parkinson's disease is characterized by **loss of dopaminergic neurons in the basal ganglia** (**[A]** substantia nigra, showing normal population of large pigmented cells; **[B]** severe depletion of pigmented cells), specifically the substantia nigra, which shows loss of pigmentation on postmortem analysis. It is usually idiopathic but may also occur after influenza infections, following carbon monoxide or manganese poisoning, after exposure to the drug **MPTP** (an impurity found in poorly synthesized heroin), with antipsychotic drugs, with basal ganglia tumors, following trauma, and after episodes of encephalitis (POSTENCEPHALITIC PARKINSONISM).
Epidemiology	A common disorder (1 per 1,000 population) that usually has an onset between 45 and 65 years of age (1 per 100 in people older than 65).
Management	**Levodopa** crosses the blood-brain barrier and is converted to dopamine in the CNS (side effects include dyskinesia, arrhythmias, nausea, vomiting, hypotension, and psychosis). It is usually administered with **carbidopa** (a dopamine decarboxylase inhibitor that does not cross the blood-brain barrier) to reduce the required dose of L-dopa and limit side effects. **Anticholinergics** are given for their beneficial effect on rigidity and tremors (side effects include dry mouth, blurring of vision, urinary retention,

PARKINSON'S DISEASE

and exacerbation of glaucoma); **amantadine** is used for mild disease, although its mechanism of action is not well understood (side effects include depression, anxiety, constipation, arrhythmias, and postural hypotension). **Bromocriptine** is a dopamine agonist associated with a lesser incidence of dyskinesia (side effects include digital vasospasm, nasal congestion, constipation, and worsening of peptic ulcer disease). **Selegiline** is an MAO-B inhibitor that prevents the breakdown of dopamine in the brain. **Surgery** includes implantation of adrenal medulla in the caudate nucleus, thalamotomy, or pallidotomy with variable results.

Complications   Progressive disability and death.

Atlas Link   U C V 1   PM-A-068

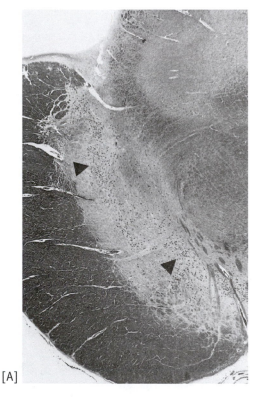

[A]

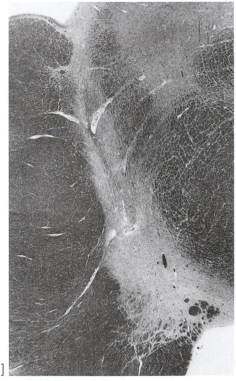

[B]

ID/CC A 65-year-old male who has been treated with **vincristine** for chronic lymphocytic leukemia complains of **tingling** (PARESTHESIAS) of the hands and feet coupled with **constipation**.

HPI The tingling began in his fingers 2 months ago with vincristine; only recently has he experienced tingling in the toes. The sensation is constant and does not change with movement or position.

PE VS: normal. PE: speech appropriate; cranial nerves intact; motor strength 5/5; DTRs 2+ except 1+ in Achilles; Babinski's absent; **decreased pinprick sensation from midfoot and wrists distally**; proprioception and vibration intact.

Labs ESR, B_{12}, folate, TSH, hemoglobin A_{1C}, and serum protein electrophoresis normal; reduction in sensory nerve action potential.

Pathogenesis Vinca alkaloids such as vincristine function as **mitotic spindle inhibitors** and interact with tubulin, resulting in the impairment of axonal transport.

Epidemiology **Vincristine** is the chemotherapeutic agent that is most commonly associated with **peripheral neuropathy**. Other common causes of drug-induced peripheral neuropathies include **cisplatin** (pure sensory neuropathy), **taxol, dapsone** (pure motor, resembles amyotrophic lateral sclerosis), **ethionamide, INH, hydralazine, phenytoin, adriamycin**, and nucleoside analogs (antiretrovirals).

Management **Reduction or withdrawal** of vincristine should result in the remission of symptoms. If motor signs are present, the drug should be stopped. If some residual paresthesia remains, symptomatic treatment can be initiated with **gabapentin** or **amitriptyline**. Stool softeners and mild cathartics may be given at the beginning of treatment.

Complications If not properly identified and if vincristine is not discontinued, the neuropathy will progress. This will result in eventual axonal damage, causing **motor weakness**. The sensory neuropathy will also worsen, extending further up the arms and legs. Acute **intestinal ileus** and **bladder neuropathies** (serious autonomic involvement) are two absolute contraindications to continued vincristine therapy.

PERIPHERAL NEUROPATHY DUE TO VINCRISTINE

ID/CC	A **65-year-old** female says that her family has noted a 1-year history of **marked personality change** and **speech difficulty**.
HPI	The patient's family claims that she is no longer interested in her hobbies of golf and reading. She now becomes angry for no apparent reason.
PE	VS: normal. PE: impaired cognitive function; CN II–XII intact; motor strength 5/5, DTRs 2+; prominent snout and grasp reflex noted.
Labs	Serum B_{12}, folate, and TSH normal. VDRL: negative.
Imaging	MR, brain: marked **bilateral frontotemporal atrophy**.
Pathogenesis	Pathologic examination reveals **atrophy** of gray and white matter in the **frontal and temporal lobes**. The characteristic lesions are argentophilic **Pick bodies**.
Management	No specific treatment. The dementia progresses over 3 to 15 years.
Complications	With progression of dementia, complications are primarily **infectious** and include aspiration pneumonia, UTIs, and decubitus ulcers.

MINICASE 263: SPINA BIFIDA

The most common developmental defect of the CNS, involving incomplete fusion of the dorsal vertebral arches and associated with inadequate folate supplementation during pregnancy
- presents as several types, ranging from spina bifida occulta, where no defect is seen and the skin is intact, to meningocele and myelomeningocele, where leptomeningeal and neural tissue may protrude through a defect in the dura mater, bone, and skin
- MR/XR show lumbar spine defect
- treat with early surgery
- complications include hydrocephalus, urinary and bowel incontinence, and lower extremity paralysis

Atlas Link: [UCV2] MC-263

PICK'S DISEASE

ID/CC	A 15-year-old Amish male presents with a 3-day history of progressive **leg weakness**.
HPI	The patient has **not had any immunizations**. His weakness has progressed such that he is now unable to climb stairs. He also complains of tingling in the legs but denies any weakness in his arms or any prior trauma.
PE	VS: fever (38.3°C); normal BP. PE: alert and oriented; CN II–XII intact; **motor tone** normal in both arms but **flaccid in both legs; motor strength 3/5 in both legs; DTRs absent bilaterally in patella and Achilles; sensory exam intact** to all primary modalities; sphincter tone normal.
Labs	CBC/LP: normal.
Pathogenesis	The causative agent of poliomyelitis is **poliovirus** serotypes 1, 2, and 3. The virus **enters the body via the GI tract** and multiplies in the lymphoid tissue of the GI tract; it then spreads to the CNS via the bloodstream, where it attacks the **motor neurons of the spinal cord** and **brainstem**. Person-to-person spread is via the oral-oral or oral-fecal route.
Epidemiology	Because of effective mass immunization, the annual incidence of polio in the United States has markedly decreased. Outbreaks occur in unimmunized individuals and in those exposed to wild-type polio virus type I.
Management	There is no specific treatment. Bed rest during the first few days reduces the risk of paralysis. Airway maintenance and ventilatory support should be instituted as necessary. Prevention with immunization is essential.
Complications	**Autonomic instability** resulting in cardiac arrhythmias and wide variation in blood pressure. Bulbar polio may jeopardize respiratory center function.

MINICASE 264: SUBARACHNOID HEMORRHAGE

Caused by aneurysm, AV malformations, or trauma
- presents as "the most severe headache of life"
- CT shows blood in cisterns and sulci
- treat with phenytoin to prevent seizures, surgical excision or embolization of aneurysm or AV malformation

Atlas Link: 🅄🅲🅥🅸 PG-P3-031

POLIOMYELITIS

ID/CC	An **18-year-old female** complains of **headache, vomiting**, and **blurred vision** for the past 2 to 3 weeks.
HPI	The patient experiences the headache as a "pressure-like" feeling in the parietal region bilaterally. She also experienced intermittent brief loss of vision while bending. She denies any associated photophobia or phonophobia.
PE	VS: normal. PE: **obese; bilateral papilledema**; neck supple; neurologic exam otherwise normal.
Labs	CBC: normal. LP: **opening pressure elevated** (34 cm H_2O); no white cells; normal protein and glucose.
Imaging	CT, head: no mass, hemorrhage, or midline shift; normal ventricle size (may even be small). MR, venography: normal (rules out transverse and sagittal sinus thrombosis).
Pathogenesis	Pseudotumor cerebri is an idiopathic condition; **overproduction of CSF** and **impairment of CSF absorption** by the arachnoid villi may be involved. Pseudotumor can follow corticosteroid withdrawal or excesses of vitamin A or tetracycline.
Epidemiology	Incidence is higher in women between the ages of 15 and 44.
Management	Withdrawal of precipitating agent. Treatment with **acetazolamide** causes decreased CSF production; if not tolerated, **furosemide** may be used. Serial LPs have a role if no medications can be tolerated. Weight loss may reduce recurrence. If visual loss continues despite medical therapy, then consider optic nerve sheath fenestration or **CSF shunting**.
Complications	**Optic atrophy** causing **permanent visual loss**; electrolyte abnormalities due to diuretic therapy.

PSEUDOTUMOR CEREBRI

ID/CC	A 50-year-old female presents with sudden-onset left-sided **facial weakness, hearing loss**, and **ear pain** of 2 days' duration.
HPI	The patient also has left-sided **throat pain**, tinnitus, vertigo, and **altered taste sensation**. She recently underwent radiation treatment for an unidentified lymphoma (immune-compromised state).
PE	**Vesicular rash** on left external ear (herpes zoster); **sensorineural hearing loss** on left side; taste absent on left anterior third of tongue; **left-sided peripheral facial palsy**.
Labs	CBC: lymphocytosis. LP: **elevated protein** in CSF. **Tzanck smear of vesicles positive**.
Imaging	CT, head: no intracranial lesions or hemorrhage.
Pathogenesis	Herpes zoster reactivation is promoted by radiation and immune compromise, including that associated with lymphoproliferative disorders, HIV, and cytotoxic chemotherapy. The virus remains dormant in nerve roots and ganglia. Herpes zoster reactivation is also called **shingles**; when it involves the **seventh and eighth cranial nerves**, it is designated Ramsay Hunt syndrome. The diagnosis of Ramsay Hunt syndrome can generally be made on the basis of history and physical exam.
Epidemiology	The incidence in children is low; in adults, it is approximately 2.5 per 1,000 per year.
Management	**Acyclovir** has been shown to reduce the duration of the vesicular rash and diminish the likelihood of postherpetic neuralgia. **Corticosteroids** may also be used as adjuvant therapy to shorten the duration and reduce the chance of postherpetic neuralgia.
Complications	Hearing loss, reactivation of virus, meningoencephalitis in immune-compromised patients.

RAMSAY HUNT SYNDROME

ID/CC   A **4-year-old girl** has been having **episodes of persistent staring** during which she does not answer questions and **looks distracted**.

HPI   One of the child's cousins has had similar episodes. During the episodes, the child rolls her eyes upward, rhythmically nods her head, and drops objects from her hand.

PE   VS: normal. PE: neurologic exam normal; with hyperventilation and under strobe light, patient was shown to have fine, twitching movements of the eyelids, pupillary dilatation (MYDRIASIS), tachycardia, and piloerection.

Labs   CBC: normal. SaO_2 98%. Lytes/LFTs/UA: normal. Calcium normal. **[A]** EEG: during seizure, **bursts of 3-cycle-per-second spike-and-wave activity** occur; in the interictal period, EEG is normal.

Imaging   CT, head: no organic pathology.

Pathogenesis   Also called **petit mal** seizures, absence seizures are inherited as an **autosomal-recessive** trait and are characterized by an

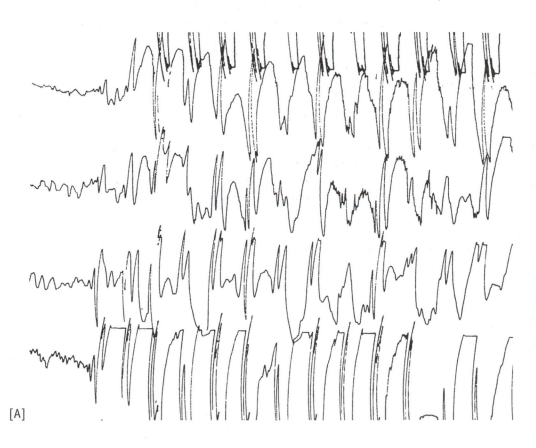

[A]

idiopathic, temporary (usually < 10 sec) **loss of awareness** that is **not preceded by an aura** and is followed by a characteristic abrupt regaining of consciousness. Hyperventilation and blinking strobe lights may precipitate the attacks.

Epidemiology **Higher incidence in children** aged 3 to 13 years; more common among girls. Petit mal seizures never begin after age 20.

Management Most patients show a **benign course**, with symptoms disappearing by puberty. **Ethosuximide** and **valproic acid** are useful drugs; a ketogenic or medium-chain triglyceride diet will also help.

Complications Loss of capacity to speak and understand with a prolonged absence seizure (PETIT MAL STATUS).

MINICASE 265: SYRINGOMYELIA

A congenital or neoplastic cystic cavity within the spinal cord that can expand in adolescents or young adults
- commonly associated with Arnold–Chiari malformation
- presents with dissociated sensory loss in a classic "capelike" distribution (shoulders and back) and flaccid upper extremity weakness with wasting of the small muscles of the hand
- presents later with spastic lower extremity weakness
- MR demonstrates the defect and differentiates from mass lesion
- treatment is rapid surgical drainage of the cyst
- complications include permanent neurologic deficits

MINICASE 266: TODD'S PARALYSIS

Postictal focal neurologic deficit
- presents with isolated limb hemiparesis that resolves over 15 to 36 hours
- no treatment is required

ID/CC	A 16-year-old **male** is brought to the physician by his mother, who reports two recent episodes during which she observed her son to be "out of it."
HPI	When he was a baby, the patient had **herpes encephalitis**. He has required remedial reading and math classes since the third grade. His episodes began when he complained of an unpleasant smell (AURA), suddenly stopped talking, and **"stared straight ahead"**; his mouth was twitching. Each episode was over in approximately 2 minutes, after which the patient was **confused and sleepy** (POSTICTAL CONFUSION). After taking a nap, he returned to normal. There is no family history of seizures, and the patient denies any alcohol or drug use.
PE	VS: normal. PE: no focal neurologic deficits.
Labs	CBC: normal. SaO_2 99%. Lytes: normal. Toxicology screen negative. EEG: normal background with **focal spike discharges over left temporal lobe**; no frank seizure activity.
Imaging	MR, brain: **left medial temporal sclerosis**.
Pathogenesis	Complex partial seizures are also referred to as **temporal lobe** or **psychomotor epilepsy**. Unlike simple partial seizures, they always involve loss of consciousness and frequently **follow auditory or olfactory auras**. Medial temporal sclerosis is a scar tissue that in this case resulted from the patient's childhood encephalitis; **scar tissue serves as a focus for seizure activity**. The cause of most seizure disorders is idiopathic, but birth injuries, head trauma, childhood febrile convulsions, and CNS malignancies can cause seizures. Seizures may occur unpredictably without any precipitating cause. However, external factors that may lower the seizure threshold include lack of sleep, missed meals, stress, alcohol or other drugs, fever, and specific stimuli such as flickering lights.
Epidemiology	Epilepsy shows a **male predominance** and is most common in the first decade of life and then after the age of 60.
Management	**Phenytoin** and **carbamazepine** are equally effective in treating complex partial seizures; the choice of drug is based on its side effect profile. The primary side effects of phenytoin are gingival hyperplasia, ataxia, lymphadenopathy, various drug interactions, hirsutism, facial coarsening, rash, and osteomalacia; those of

carbamazepine are leukopenia, nausea, vomiting, and hepatotoxicity.

Complications   **Secondary generalization** of seizure that began as a complex partial seizure; serious injury during seizure episode; and **status epilepticus**.

MINICASE 267: RESTRAINTS

Restraints are defined as any physical or pharmacologic means used to restrict a patient's movement, activity, or access to his or her body
- patients may be restrained only if it is absolutely necessary to treat their medical symptoms or to prevent them from harming themselves or others
- restraining patients raises many medicoethical and medicolegal issues, such as infringement on patient autonomy, limitations on freedom of movement, claims of battery, and risk of physical or psychological injury from restraints
- the use of restraints must be consistent with federal and state laws, hospital regulations, JCAHO requirements, and, most significantly, sound clinical judgment

---

MINICASE 268: PSEUDOSEIZURES

Causes include malingering, part of conversion disorder
- presents with seizure that stops with abrupt commands and blepharospasm that occurs during examination of pupils, and patient's hand not dropping onto face if dropped from straight above
- EEG normal
- refer to psychiatry

MINICASE 269: PSEUDODEMENTIA

A cognitive dysfunction resulting from depression
- reversible and common
- positive screen for depression
- treat with SSRIs

ID/CC	A **10-month-old child** is rushed to the emergency room because of sudden loss of consciousness, rigidity of muscles followed by **jerky movements of all limbs, upward rolling of the eyes, and urination**.
HPI	The patient was being treated for **severe otitis media** and had a 40.2°C temperature when the seizure began.
PE	VS: **fever** (38.1°C). PE: neck supple; pupils equal, round, and reactive to light; no focal neurologic signs; severe otitis media in right ear.
Labs	CBC: leukocytosis with left shift. SaO$_2$ 98%. Lytes/UA: normal. LP: CSF normal. EEG: posterior asymmetric slowing of background.
Imaging	CT, brain: normal.
Pathogenesis	Febrile seizures are those that occur in children **younger than 5 years** and **older than 3 months of age**, have **no organic cause**, and are **precipitated by a high fever**.
Epidemiology	There is usually a family history of the disease, and recurrence occurs in 30% of patients.
Management	**Temperature control with acetaminophen** and cold baths. **Diazepam** may be used in the acute setting to control seizures. Treat the precipitating illness with appropriate antibiotics.
Complications	**Recurrence** (occurs more often in those with a young age at onset, those with a family history, those with seizures at a lower temperature level, and children with marked slowing on EEG), mental deficiency, **developmental disturbances** (more so in patients with previous neurologic disturbance and with focal seizures), status epilepticus, and epilepsy development (rare).

ID/CC A 16-year-old male presents with sudden **loss of consciousness** and muscle hypertonia followed by **rhythmic movements of the limbs** with upward rolling of the eyes, tongue biting, and urinary incontinence; he is now in a state of confusion and lethargy.

HPI He is otherwise healthy and is a good student. He has two cousins who suffer from a seizure disorder. He does not take any illicit drugs or medications.

PE VS: normal. PE: lethargic; complains of headache but is awake and oriented; no cyanosis; lesion on anterior third of tongue attributed to bite during seizure; nonfocal neurologic examination.

Labs CBC/LFTs: normal. SaO_2 99%. Lytes: normal. UA: toxicology screen negative. **Prolactin elevated** (it does not rise after a psychogenic tonic-clonic "seizure"). ECG: normal sinus rhythm. **[A]** EEG: diffuse slowing with generalized spike-and-wave pattern. LP: CSF normal.

Imaging CT, head: no apparent intracranial pathology.

Pathogenesis Grand mal seizures are also called generalized tonic-clonic seizures. A tonic-clonic seizure can begin as a partial complex seizure, in which case it is termed partial complex seizure secondarily generalized.

Epidemiology Half of patients who suffer a new-onset tonic-clonic seizure will have a recurrence. Epilepsy may remit spontaneously in up to one-third of cases and may be controlled with medications.

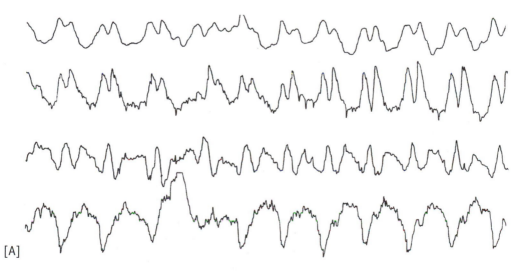

[A]

SEIZURE, GRAND MAL

Management   Start with a low dose of valproic **acid** (side effects include severe, fatal hepatotoxicity, pancreatitis, thrombocytopenia, hair loss, GI upset, ataxia, sedation, and tremors) and increase dosage slowly; the vast majority of cases can be controlled with a single drug. If not effective despite therapeutic blood levels, the addition of **phenytoin** (side effects include numerous drug interactions, gingival hyperplasia, facial coarsening, ataxia, hirsutism, rash, lymphadenopathy, megaloblastic anemia, and osteomalacia), **phenobarbital** (side effects include sedation, depression, and numerous drug interactions), **carbamazepine** (side effects include GI upset, thrombocytopenia, aplastic anemia, hepatotoxicity, ataxia, vertigo, and diplopia), or primidone (main side effect is sedation) may be helpful. When the patient has been seizure free on medications for 2 years, tapering may be attempted with the knowledge that recurrence is likely.

Complications   **Chronicity**, difficulty controlling seizure activity, **status epilepticus** (single seizure lasting > 30 minutes or a series of seizures with no return to consciousness lasting > 30 minutes), and **motor vehicle accidents**.

ID/CC   A 66-year-old male with **lung cancer** is discovered **"shaking"** in bed and unable to speak.

HPI   The patient was diagnosed with lung cancer 6 months ago and has been treated with chemotherapy. He has complained of severe early-morning **headaches** associated with **nausea and projectile vomiting**, which improve as the day progresses, coupled with **blurred vision** (due to papilledema). Now he is **confused**, but his right arm and leg are no longer shaking.

PE   VS: normal. PE: drowsy but able to follow commands; **4/5 strength in right** arm and leg with 5/5 strength on left; **bilateral papilledema**.

Labs   CBC: anemia. SaO_2 97%. Lytes: normal. Troponin I normal.

Imaging   **[A]** CT, head (with contrast): **ring-enhancing lesion** (1) in the **left parietal region** with surrounding mild edema.

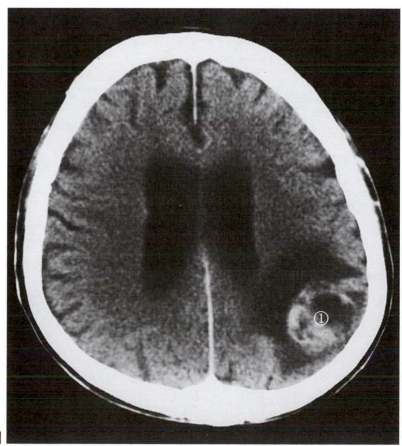

[A]

SEIZURE, METASTATIC DISEASE

Pathogenesis The metastatic lesion serves as the seizure focus. Symptoms are due to edema surrounding the mass and destruction of brain tissue by the metastases.

Epidemiology Fifteen percent of patients with diagnosed cancer develop cerebral metastases (40% are single lesions). **Malignancies that metastasize to the brain** are **lung, breast, melanoma, renal cell**, and **colon**.

Management Administer **lifelong antiepileptic treatment (phenytoin)**; obtain an MR of the brain to determine the possible presence of one or more metastatic lesions. In the presence of a **single brain lesion** and if the patient is in relatively good health, **resection** will improve life span. If the patient is in poor health or has **multiple metastatic lesions** of the brain, then **radiation** (breast and small cell lung cancer metastases respond well; melanoma and kidney adenocarcinoma metastases are resistant to radiotherapy) and **steroids** (IV dexamethasone) should be used to reduce the edema surrounding the lesion.

Complications Recurrent seizures (due to scarring or to persistence or further growth of tumor), severe headaches, altered mental status, and increasing neurologic deficits.

ID/CC   A **32-year-old male** fell two stories from the roof of a house and is now **unable to get up or move his legs**.

HPI   The patient was previously healthy.

PE   VS: normal. PE: able to follow commands; speech appropriate; cranial nerves intact; 5/5 strength in upper extremities; **0/5 motor strength in lower extremities**; DTRs 2+ in upper extremities; DTRs absent in lower extremities (may increase later); **no sensation to pinprick below iliac crest** (T12 sensory level); **rectal tone markedly diminished**.

Imaging   MR, spine: fracture-dislocation of the T12 vertebral body with compression of the spinal cord (the majority of thoracolumbar fractures occur between T12 and L2).

Pathogenesis   There are **four types** of spinal injury: flexion, extension, axial due to compressive force, and rotational. Spinal cord injury can result in neurogenic shock, when the sympathetic innervation to the vasculature is compromised; patients experience hypotension and bradycardia.

Epidemiology   **Younger men** are at highest risk. Associated with a mortality rate of 5% to 20%; quadriplegia is the end result in 30% to 40% of cases.

Management   ABCs; **mechanical** stabilization of the entire spine to prevent further injury. Administer **IV methylprednisolone** within 24 hours of injury to minimize edema. **Surgery** should be conducted for permanent stabilization of the spine, and baclofen given for muscle spasms. Intermittent straight catheterization due to urinary incontinence. Insertion of nasogastric tube.

Complications   Autonomic dysfunction, respiratory and skin infections due to immobility, urinary incontinence, UTIs, painful muscle spasms, and constipation requiring daily bowel regimen (stool softener, enemas).

SPINAL CORD INJURY

ID/CC	An **8-year-old boy** presents with **"jerking" movements**.

HPI	The boy has no significant medical history and does not have a regular pediatrician. His mother cannot remember if his vaccinations are up to date. He had **measles at 10 months of age** but has developed normally. In the last month, his grades at school have worsened considerably. Two days ago, his mother noted the onset of continuous "jerking" movements.

PE	VS: normal. PE: **lethargic** but able to cooperate; neck supple; cranial nerves intact; motor tone exceptional given continuous **myoclonic movements** involving all four extremities; DTRs 2+ and symmetric throughout; finger-to-nose exam reveals mild **dysmetria**; gait normal; sensation intact to pinprick in all four extremities.

Labs	CBC: normal. EEG: **burst suppression**. LP: normal opening pressure; normal protein and glucose with no white cells; CSF antibody titer **elevated** for **measles-specific antibodies**. No organisms on Gram stain; **elevated oligoclonal bands**.

Imaging	CT, brain: cerebral edema and diffuse hypodense signal in white matter bilaterally.

Pathogenesis	Due to **accumulation of defective measles virus in neurons**. In those with subacute sclerosing panencephalitis (SSPE), neurons contain viral nucleic acid and proteins that cannot be integrated into viral particles. SSPE is characterized by **three clinical stages**: stage I is marked by behavioral and cognitive decline, stage II by motor dysfunction (spasticity, weakness) and often myoclonic jerks and seizures, and stage III by stupor, coma, and autonomic failure (loss of thermoregulation). Death occurs 1 to 3 years after onset of symptoms.

Epidemiology	Fewer than 10 cases per year in the United States. Average age of onset is 6 to 8 years; the median interval between acute measles infection and SSPE is 8 years. **Males** are affected three times more often than females. Large-scale measles vaccination programs have resulted in a 20-fold decrease in the risk of SSPE.

Management	**Supportive care**; antiepileptic treatment if seizures occur.

Complications	Seizures, autonomic failure, coma, and death.

SUBACUTE SCLEROSING PANENCEPHALITIS

ID/CC A **70-year-old woman** presents with a **severe, intermittent right temporal headache** and **fever** of 2 months' duration and **blurred vision in the right eye** for 2 days.

HPI The headache is neither relieved nor aggravated by changes in position or activity level. The patient also complains of **pain in the jaw when chewing** (CLAUDICATION), weight loss, and discomfort on combing the right scalp but denies any associated nausea, vomiting, photophobia, or phonophobia. She has achieved some relief with acetaminophen.

PE VS: mild fever; otherwise normal. PE: visual acuity normal; funduscopy reveals a swollen right disk; palpation reveals a right **temporal artery** that is **tender, pulseless, nodular**, and tortuous; locally tender scalp.

Labs CBC: mild normocytic, normochromic **anemia**; mild leukocytosis and thrombocytosis. **Markedly elevated ESR** and acute phase reactants (C1-reactive protein); serum protein electrophoresis reveals mild polyclonal hypergammaglobulinemia; rheumatoid factor, ANA, and dsDNA negative (rules out connective tissue disorders); **temporal artery biopsy reveals mononuclear cell infiltrates in the media**, particularly in the internal elastic lamina, as well as intimal thickening and granulomas containing multinucleated giant cells, histiocytes, and lymphocytes.

Pathogenesis The etiology of temporal arteritis is unknown. The histopathologic lesion is **giant-cell granuloma** within the vessel wall, leading to stenosis of the lumen. Involvement of an affected artery is patchy. Vascular inflammation is found most often in the superficial temporal arteries as well as in the vertebral, ophthalmic, and posterior ciliary arteries.

Epidemiology Median age of onset is 75. More prevalent in females.

Management **High-dose corticosteroids urgently** to prevent blindness; continue until symptoms resolve and ESR normalizes, and then taper slowly. Early temporal artery biopsy yields a definitive diagnosis. Most patients require a minimum of 1 to 2 years of therapy; some will require chronic steroid administration.

TEMPORAL ARTERITIS (GIANT CELL ARTERITIS)

Complications   Complications include loss of vision and opportunistic infections (due to long-term prednisone treatment). Death may occur from strokes, ruptured aorta secondary to aortitis, and MI from coronary arteritis.

Atlas Link   ⬛UCV1⬛ PM-P3-034

ID/CC	A 62-year-old housewife complains of **recurrent episodes of headaches** that she has experienced since the age of 40.
HPI	Initially her headaches presented as a moderate **squeezing pain** in the **bilateral frontal area**. The headaches occurred twice monthly and were relieved with two acetaminophen tablets and a nap. For the past two years, the headaches have occurred three to four times a week, with accompanying nausea approximately one to two times a week. Minimal relief is obtained with ibuprofen. She denies associated phonophobia, photophobia, or focal motor deficits.
PE	VS: normal. PE: funduscopic exam reveals sharp disks bilaterally; visual acuity 20/20 bilaterally; neurologic exam normal.
Labs	ESR: normal.
Imaging	CT, head: no intracranial lesions or hemorrhage.
Pathogenesis	Overuse of OTC medications or depression may play a role. Chronic tension headache is characterized by pain that is **bilateral** in location and present for **more than 15 days per month** for at least the last **6 months**; it may or may not be accompanied by nausea, and there is no vomiting or photophobia. Pain is rarely throbbing in nature and is not aggravated by routine physical activity.
Management	Add **amitriptyline** or gabapentin **to NSAIDs** or **acetaminophen**. Four to six weeks of treatment is necessary to determine efficacy.
Complications	Recurrent headaches.

TENSION HEADACHE

ID/CC	A **47-year-old** male complains of episodes of severe **pain in the right cheek** over the past year.
HPI	The pain is **electric in character** and **occurs while he is shaving**. Each episode lasts 2 to 4 minutes. At first, the episodes occurred daily for 3 to 4 days and then disappeared for 2 months. For the past 3 weeks, the pain has occurred every day.
PE	VS: normal. PE: mild touch in **right V2** (maxillary subdivision of trigeminal) **distribution** reproduces the painful episode; remainder of neurologic exam normal.
Labs	ESR: normal.
Imaging	MR, brain: normal.
Pathogenesis	Trigeminal neuralgia is usually **idiopathic**, but may be caused by a meningioma that compresses the gasserian ganglion, by a schwannoma of the nerve, by malignant infiltration of the skull base, or by herpes zoster infection. V2 or V3 distributions are more commonly affected than V1. The typical course is relapsing/remitting over several years.
Epidemiology	Ninety percent of patients are **older than 40 years**.
Management	**Carbamazepine**, gabapentin, **phenytoin**, or baclofen. If the patient fails medical treatment, then multiple **surgical treatments** are available, including alcohol block of the branch of the trigeminal nerve that is painful as well as percutaneous thermocoagulation of the trigeminal nerve sensory root (the procedure of choice in the elderly).

ID/CC A 31-year-old female presents with **headaches, nausea, and vomiting** of 2 months' duration.

HPI The headaches have slowly increased in severity over the past month. She denies any change in vision or motor weakness. Her **mother died of cancer** at the age of 28.

PE VS: normal. PE: speech appropriate; mild papilledema in right disk; left disk not well visualized owing to **enlarged globular blood vessel** (HAMARTOMA); finger-to-nose exam significant for mild **dysmetria**; gait slightly **wide-based**; tandem gait severely impaired; sensory exam intact.

Labs CBC: **polycythemia** (due to ectopic erythropoietin production by hemangioblastoma).

Imaging CT, brain: large, low-density, **cystic-appearing mass** in the midline of the **cerebellum**. CT, abdomen: multiple **bilateral renal cysts**.

Pathogenesis Von Hippel–Lindau disease is characterized by cerebellar **hemangioblastomas** or **retinal angiomas** and by the presence of **cysts in at least one visceral organ**. Within the same family, all gradations of the syndrome may be found. The gene locus for von Hippel-Lindau syndrome has been mapped to **chromosome 3p**.

Epidemiology Becomes symptomatic during adult life and has an **autosomal-dominant** pattern of inheritance.

Management **Surgical excision** of hemangioblastomas (surgical approach aided by cerebral angiogram). Annual ophthalmologic exams to screen for **retinal hemangioblastoma**.

Complications Retinal hemangioblastoma, recurrence of hemangioblastoma, adrenal abnormalities (pheochromocytoma, adrenal medulla cyst, adrenal cortical hyperplasia), and renal carcinoma.

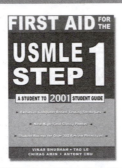
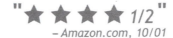
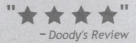
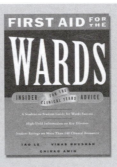
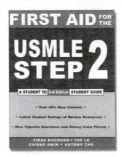
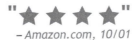
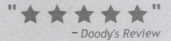
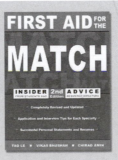